NUTRIGENOMICS

BIOHACKING FOR A BETTER YOU

BY: KUSHA KARVANDI

The creator of

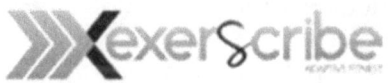

Exerscribe.com

Publishing services provided by 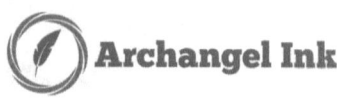 **Archangel Ink**

ISBN: 1517740754
ISBN-13: 978-1517740757

Introduction

If you're reading this book, it's because you're at a crossroads. You've tried everything, but you still haven't achieved the health and body you desire.

You've counted endless calories and popped fistfuls of vitamins and supplements, and yet you still aren't getting anywhere. Meanwhile, you see others do virtually no exercise, eat bad food, and still look great. We call them genetically blessed, lucky, or some combination of the two.

But what about you?

You're left still wondering about your own health & fitness goals and probably getting pretty ticked off by the fact that you've tried every diet, fad, and supplement that you've been told will make you lose weight and improve your life.

I bring up this scenario for two reasons. The first is because I want you to be very clear about something. If you've been proactive to achieve health and haven't seen results, then it's safe to say that the problem isn't that you're not doing enough. The second reason is because if this type of situation applies to you, then there is definitely something working against your body. My goal is to help you pinpoint the root issue so that you can solve it and reach your maximum quality of health.

I'm not talking about another health gimmick, diet, or exercise program that's "guaranteed" to shed the weight. If you're looking for that type of program, you're going to be sorely disappointed because it simply doesn't exist. Perhaps you don't agree with me. Maybe you've followed the results of amazing diet plans and you read the reviews of so many satisfied people. Let's consider this idea for a moment. Out of all those people who claim a program worked for them, say 100 people claiming these amazing results, there might be 10 to 20 who don't receive results. 80% to 90% is a great thing to claim, right? If you belong in that group, then it's absolutely a great thing.

But what about the 10% to 20%? What happens to them?

There has to be some hope for those who fall into the treacherous 20%, right? Well, first of all, the reality is that this 20% group is more like 90% due to embellished success stories and weight gain relapses. Second, this book WILL help you find the long-term solution that will work for you. No more fad diets, calorie counting, or food logging. Only sustainable strategies that fit into your lifestyle.

I believe that everyone deserves a chance to be healthy, fit, and lean. But health is more than a series of diets and exercise plans. It's a science that can change your body if you understand it.

My wife and I have written another book called *Nutriscribe*. In that book, we discuss food and metabolism from a general understanding of the body. We also discuss guidelines for fat loss, athletic conditioning, and some other general dietary information. This book is written to supplement the information in that book in an effort to give you the best, well-rounded collection on the topic of food, nutrition, your body, and your health.

Chapter 1

The Truth about Genes

In this first chapter, I am going to reveal to you why you have more control over your genes and your body than you think do. Most people believe their genes are "set in stone" and unchangeable, but the truth is your perception and environment can actually influence your DNA to work for your rather than against you.

From our youth we've been pestered by the dogma that our biology dictates our outcomes; that our DNA and genes are responsible for our misfortunes in health and our abundance. But that couldn't be further from the truth.

I don't blame society or the media. I blame science.

If you recall from the history books, centuries ago, religion ranked highest in being able to explain things. And then we hit this turning point. Science took a sharp left while religion went right. People like Isaac Newton and Charles Darwin entered the scene and made a name for themselves in their explanation of physical matter.

These early scientists grounded their theories on the premise that religion focused too much on the invisible and not enough on the visible. So they settled on the assumption that the invisible stuff didn't matter. Energy? What's that? Proteins? We don't care about those either.

Fast forward to the 20th Century, and that dogma still exists. In fact, it's more prevalent than ever before. And guess where it took the greatest foothold? Modern medicine.

Like Newton and Darwin, our modern scientists wanted to understand nature so that they could control it, dominate it, which was a stark contrast to what science aspired to previously, where they sought to understand nature to better live in harmony with it. So what better place to start than the human body, a machine so complex it must hold all the secrets of the cosmos. I agree that somewhere deep within us lies a powerful binary (computer geek talk for code) that can unlock tremendous potential.

The problem with the human body is that it's too complex, so scientists went a few layers deeper and settled on the cell. They figured that since our bodies are composed of 50-75 trillion of these cells, it must be the perfect place to start the conquest. As they studied cells, they tried to find similarities between their parts and structures and us.

And then they found something astonishing. The nucleus. The nucleus of the cells contained the DNA, genes, and chromosomes, and they believed this structure was the "brain" of the cell. Just like our brain tells our body what to do, they were certain that the nucleus told the cell what to do. This, as you may have guessed, is how DNA became culpable for our shortcomings.

Interestingly enough, all of this was disproven. See, for the nucleus to truly be the "brain" of the cell, the cell would not be able to survive without it. However, when they removed the nucleus from the cell, it lived! This is where the truth bomb hits. The nucleus (and your genes) never controlled the cell. It was the cell membrane.

The cell membrane encapsulates the cell, separating the interior of the cell from the environment. On the surface of the cell membrane are receptors, little antennas that are constantly seeking a signal from the environment. When that signal arrives, it binds to the receptor, which then activates a protein. This protein, like all proteins in the cell, is composed of specific building blocks known as amino acids. The tail ends of the amino acids are oppositely charged (in terms of electrons) before being activated. Just like a magnet, when the protein is sitting inactive in the cell with oppositely charged tails, it sits in the most stable conformation, which is where the tails are nearest each other (because opposites attract).

This may sound like a lot of scientific jargon, but it is actually very important because it proves that changes to our bodies (such as body fat storage, disease, etc.) occur from the outside in rather than the inside out like most people believe.

After an environmental signal makes its way into the cell (via the receptor), a chain reaction occurs that changes the electron charge of one of the amino acid tails and essentially turns that inactive protein "on." This gets the protein moving since the two tails are no longer oppositely charged and trying to move away from each other to make the protein more stable. Then, like a bucket brigade at a forest fire, the protein passes the charge to the next protein, which passes it to the next and so forth. This often creates a second reaction in the cell, which takes place at the nucleus.

Since the DNA lives in the nucleus, you can see how your environment influences your DNA (such as how eating processed carbs and sugars can lead to obesity, diabetes, and even cancer).

Our DNA is unique and composed of strands of genes. These genes are covered in protein sleeves. When that secondary reaction occurs, it removes the protein sleeve and exposes the gene strand so that it can be expressed. As I said earlier, we realized the nucleus was not the brain of the cell but instead a copy machine. The cell has several parts that break down and must be replaced. The genes provide the blueprints for the RNA (aka the copier) to then copy and regenerate needed parts.

Again, if you haven't realized already, what I've just proven to you is that your genes do NOT dictate your outcomes. It is your environment.

Remember, your environment provides the signal that your cell membrane then interprets and decides what behavior will be required. Sounds familiar, huh? As human beings, we do the exact same thing, and we call it perception. External influences from our environment are so powerful that they get embedded deep in our thoughts, behaviors, habits, and beliefs.

In the 1960s, Dr. Bruce Lipton did studies on stem cells (way before it was cool) and proved something remarkable. When he put the stem cells in different culture mediums, they all harvested something different even though the cells (and, more importantly, the genes in those cells) were the same. One petri dish harvested muscle tissue, one fat, one bone.

It's extremely important that you pay attention to this because this is where it all comes together. The only difference between those petri dishes was the culture mediums—the environments. Now, you need to think of your thoughts as electric impulses. These impulses can trigger chemical changes to your blood. Like a cell membrane, your skin separates all of what's inside you from the outside world. So, if we think of your skin as a giant petri dish, your blood as the culture medium, and the 50-75 trillion cells inside as the stem cells, what do you think happens when your thought impulses influence the chemical makeup of your culture medium (aka blood)?

Now you're getting it. The funny thing is that we knew all along that the chromosomes weren't alone. They weren't just a bunch of DNA and genetic strands. There are proteins present in your chromosomes too. And not just a few proteins; we're talking nearly fifty percent of the composition of your chromosomes. You'd think scientists would have been less careless than to just toss out half our chromosomes during research, but it wasn't their fault entirely. They were trapped by old dogma. When most of the major studies were done, the proteins were not as visible as the DNA and genes. And since they were taught to discard the invisible, they did.

It all makes perfect sense now, doesn't it?

Just because you may have an obesity "gene" in your family history doesn't mean you will be obese. That gene has to be expressed, and, specifically, it needs an environmental signal to be "turned on." We know this is true because if you had a cancer "gene," it would be expressing itself from birth, metastasizing immediately. But we know that's not the case. In this book, I'm going to show you how you can get food to work for you by turning the right genes on and the wrong ones off.

You know, it used to be that if someone was overweight, people figured they ate too much, were lazy, and didn't exercise. That archaic way of approaching fitness morphed into the concept of overeating, or simply eating too much of the wrong stuff. This latter thought birthed the idea of calorie counting.

Millions saw extreme weight loss when they started counting calories, but others were still not convinced they had discovered the driving factor behind fitness. That's because people started to realize that weight wasn't the only factor when it came to fitness. There were also health levels that needed to be considered. How prone are you to sickness? Are you tired often without any explanation as to why?

People found that even if they were losing weight, their overall health and fitness levels may not have been improving.

The field of nutrigenomics, or the study of nutrition on genomic expression, has received significant attention recently for its potential to prevent, eliminate, or treat chronic illness and even certain cancers. In other words, through small but highly specific and informative dietary changes you can massively affect your nutrition and overall health. I'm sure that you've heard "you are what you eat." Well, just how true is that? Before we can get into the role that nutrition plays in your body's health and nutrition levels, we must first take a look at what genes are.

What Are Genes?

Genes hold the code to make the proteins our body needs to operate. In its simplest definition, genes are our DNA. Proteins are needed to access energy and perform a variety of daily activities, including walking, running, and exercising. If your protein isn't being metabolized (or broken down for bodily usage) appropriately, the effect can be like going to the gym and exercising daily while steadily getting worse in performance and physique. There are many people who experience this.

Gene Regulation

Aside from building new protein for our body's consumption, genes also regulate our human features such as hair color (lush solid colors or early thinning and gray hair sightings), body fat distribution, and muscle mass. The gene code that regulates these physical attributes can actually be switched on and off and sometimes even suppressed through a process called gene regulation. This is where nutrigenomics gets interesting. Certain genes, when either suppressed, turned off, or turned on, can determine things such as hair color in adulthood, but also your weight, immunity tolerance, and even protection from cancer and other diseases.

The code expressed or suppressed in your genes is affected naturally through different stages of development such as childhood, adolescence, and adulthood. Up until recently, scientists weren't very concerned about this part of gene regulation. Scientists tried to provide an explanation of most maladaptive gene expression from internal influences, instead of acknowledging the role of the environment on gene expression and our ability to adapt.

Hormones, genetic mutations, and environmental exposure can cause unintended effects on gene regulation. To explain these different areas, I could get into some pretty detailed scientific talk—but you're not scientists. You're interested in your health and nutrition, and I want to focus on gene expression solely from this angle because that's my area of expertise.

Genetic Mutations

Oftentimes, the word "mutation" is thought to be something more horrific than it really is. In your gene code, if any part is repeated, deleted, or missing, the code has been mutated. Mutations can't spontaneously create new information (such as new body parts) but simply alter the code for what already exists.

If we use cancerous tumor cells as an example, the tumor cells were likely generated from a disruption in your genetic expression. You actually have genetic control mechanisms such as DNA methylation (methylation deactivates genes) that, when expressed, will prevent the growth and metastasis of cancerous tumors. However, if your DNA is demethylated from poor diet, stress, environmental factors, etc., your natural genetic control mechanisms cannot do their job to effectively protect you. So when your health is poor, DNA demethylation is working against you by turning the harmful genetic switches "on". Conversely, when health is optimal DNA methylation turns the adverse genetic switches "off".

In this scenario, which is quite common due to the standard American lifestyle, your cells are reading the blueprints (aka your genes) incorrectly. It's as if the RNA (the copy machine of the cell) is reading your blueprints (genes) upside-down. This leads to genetic mutations such as cancerous tumors.

Hormones

The best example of this that I can give is with steroids. We can tell when athletes are using steroids because their physiques dramatically change, often rapidly. I'll be blunt about it: men grow breasts and women lose theirs. Men start to take on feminine features while women take on more masculine qualities. To this day, steroids are our most significant example of how hormones control gene expression.

Environmental Exposure

Environmental exposure is one of the more significant ways that gene expression is influenced. Although there are many different factors at play, environmental exposure is something we can control. For example, men and women can develop dangerously high levels of estrogen through various everyday products they use, including plastics and personal skin care items. Other environmental factors include air quality, dust, allergens, light, and electronics. Later in the book, we will cover some tactics to eradicate these issues.

Nutrigenomics & Fitness

When it comes to fitness, you can't rely on exercise alone. I'm sure you've heard the saying "You can't exercise your way out of a bad diet." Nutrigenomics, however, is more than just eating better; it's about gaining precision with your diet and supplementation so that you're maximizing the expression of the right genes while minimizing the expression of the wrong ones. When you have this kind of precision, you're no longer guessing. And your "fitness" will become less about vanity and will instead pervade and optimize more important areas of your life like your relationships, career, and happiness.

So how exactly do nutrigenomics, fitness, and optimal health work together? Over the remainder of the book, this is the question that we're going to answer. When people start sprouting an interest in fitness and health, it's usually because they want to know two things: how to drop fat and how to gain muscle. Of course, these people don't want to look like crap or feel miserable in the process. They want to look great and feel great, too! In health and fitness, I consider them to be the same thing, and by the time we're done with this book, you'll know how to have both.

Chapter 2

Stress

The brain is often associated with something called the central nervous system (CNS). The CNS is like the motherboard of a computer—it tells every organ what to do. But I like to think of things differently. Instead, I like to think of it as the "extended nervous system," which consists primarily of the brain, skin, and digestive system. If you look at all the major health problems out there, they're not being caused by high blood pressure or high cholesterol—it's stress. I'm not talking about just mental stress; I'm referring to postural and digestive stress as well.

When you sit all day long and eat junk food (don't tell me you eat "clean," either, until after you finish this book), you create stress in the body. We won't go into your postural stressors, but if you want to begin reversing the damage, try our workouts via the Exerscribe app. Our warm-ups and workouts are designed to give you a "neural reset" and robust foundation for building some lean muscle and strength.

Now let's talk about the stress on your digestive system. Your immune system, for example, is built by your gut flora (proper balance of beneficial bacteria), not white blood cells. We've been led to believe the opposite since childhood, but the reality is that your gut health is your immune system, and the other mechanisms are really just emergency response systems. When you eat a diet balanced in fat-soluble vitamins, minerals, enzymes, high-quality proteins, and plant matter, your brain and body function at their apex. Yes, this means you need saturated fat in your diet. But before you go eating a brick of butter, let me explain something fundamental: quality matters.

There is a distinct difference in how your body responds to butter from cows that were grass-fed vs. butter from grain-fed cows. The latter is stripped of many fat-soluble vitamins, minerals, cofactors, and enzymes (such as lipase, an enzyme that helps break down fatty acids). Processing makes this low-quality form of saturated fat weaker and less stable than its grass-fed counterpart.

When you consume cholesterol from unstable saturated fats like cheap butter, margarine, canola oil, and other hydrogenated vegetable oils and trans fats, this cholesterol easily oxidizes in the body (think of oxidation like rust in the body). This oxidation creates further stress in the body, which leads to a cascade of dysfunction and problems such as diabetes, arterial plaque, and heart disease.

One of the best ways to correct this problem is to eliminate the artificial, processed fats and carbs and replace them with natural sources. The next step is to create balance. You want most of your fat intake to come from saturated fat (e.g., butter from grass-fed cows) and monounsaturated fat (e.g., avocado and coconut oil), and very small portion from polyunsaturated fat (e.g.,fish oil and olive oil).

The third step is to trade your grains for green vegetables when possible (don't be afraid of fruit either). The fourth step is to try to get more high-quality, protein-dense foods at each meal (typically one to two palm-sized servings). And the last step is to practice eating to "80% full."

If you practice those habits, you'll have an excellent platform for biohacking your DNA and genetic potential. Unfortunately, most people don't consider this concept and try all kinds of supplements and diet fads to no avail because they didn't fix their bad habits. What you need to realize is that your poor habits are working against you to turn the wrong genes on. But, like I said, we can turn the wrong genes off by following the five habits I mentioned above, and by introducing some new things that I'll get to in a bit.

Chapter 3

Genetic Switches

Alright, at the risk of making you feel like you've gone back to high school to talk genes and proteins, I'm going to explain and define genetic switches. Just like I couldn't move forward without first explaining gene regulation and covering nutrigenomics, I can't push on without covering this topic. I'd like to start with the simple definition first:

Genetic Switch: *A genetic switch is one of the many different proteins that can bind to DNA, causing the alteration of how a specific gene is expressed. In effect, the action of protein binding to a gene is like a specific gene being switched on and off, like a light.*

Essentially, your genes control the information that can help boost your metabolism, slow it down, drop fat, or store it up. Clearly, when it comes to nutrigenomics, what you want to do is get your genes expressing the good and switching off the bad.

How It Works

The body is a complicated mess, if you ask me. It seems that it would be so much easier if our bodies had a clear-cut list of instructions for us to follow in order to achieve optimum health. Unfortunately, they just don't. That's why so many people bounce from one fad to another. Nutrigenomics is promising because it helps organize our individuality into an array of specific markers (e.g., gut biome, amino acids, fatty acids, etc.), which can be used to create a unique plan for diet and supplementation. Instead of popping another prescription the doctor arbitrarily prescribed (or misprescribed due to misdiagnosis), you can spend a little more time getting a thorough evaluation of your genetic markers so that you can improve your health with nature's medicine–food.

Although the study of nutrigenomics and how nutrition affects gene expression is a relatively new field of study, the concept has been around for decades. Epigenetics, the study of how certain genes are turned "on" or "off," has been studied since the 1960s. Scientists have been able to determine that there are three ways our genes can be switched on and off. In order to grasp what's best for your body, we're going to discuss all three.

Gene Transcription

This is the natural way that genes are given the instructions for their replication, or copying, behavior. When genes are transcribed, code is written that tells them to stop production and/or increase or lower their activity. During transcription, the original gene sequence within the cell nucleus makes a copy. That copy is the transcription.

I want you to think of the transcription process like a copy machine. When the copy machine is fed the document properly and is working properly, it makes perfect copies. However, if something goes wrong in this process such as the paper gets jammed, the document is inserted and read upside-down, or the copy machine gets a bug, the copy generated will be very poor, if not something entirely unintended.

When the messenger, called mRNA (messenger ribonucleic acid), carrying the directions to create new protein leaves the cell, an external signal (a protein called the transcription factor) can get in the way and completely cover up the directions.

Transcription Factor & Translation

Once mRNA is carrying the transcription, it must first translate, or decode, the transcription (copy) of genes. Transcription factors bind to DNA, blocking, suppressing, hiding, or promoting how the code is translated or read. It's important to realize that these factors are not evil. They're found in about 8% of the genes within the human genome.

They're there to help regulate the life cycle within us, as well as in all other forms of life. When these factors are working properly, they correctly facilitate the growth from infant to toddler to young child to teen to adult and throughout time until death. It is when these factors are corrupted or mutated that we have a problem. Later on, we'll discuss what causes the corruption or mutation.

Nutrigenomics—How does what you eat affect genetic expression?

You probably know that we can't change our genes—before birth, each of us has a unique pattern of thymine, alanine, cytosine, and guanine that essentially makes us who we are. After all, we commonly hear people attribute certain issues or difficulties to genetics. And it's true that certain disorders are inherited and can't (yet) be altered.

A common misconception, however, is that the fact that genes are unchangeable means they are always expressed the same way. This is emphatically untrue. There are many environmental factors that can affect gene expression, whether they're beneficial or not. Many genes can have their expression changed due to environmental factors. And one of the lesser-known factors that can have this affect is diet. We all know that diet can affect body composition, as certain diets and supplements can result in weight loss or gain, addition of muscle, and loss of fat, etc. But even vitamins found in a typical, non-supplemented diet can impact genetic expression.

The study of the impact of diet and environment on genetics is a well-known science. Nutrigenomics refers to the impact nutrition has on genetic expression, while epigenetics refers to the study of environment and its effect of gene expression.

Before delving into the importance of vitamins and supplements to gene expression, though, it's necessary to understand the basics of DNA methylation and its connection to gene expression and gene silencing.

Mechanism of Action – Diet and DNA Methylation and Gene Expression

The idea of foods and other supplements altering gene expression may sound foreign, but when you look at the actual mechanism behind it, it becomes more logical.

Certain supplements alter genetic expression by virtue of their ability to methylate DNA. Methylation refers to the addition of a methyl group (CH3) to a base (cytosine, guanine, thymine, or alanine). Appropriately methylated tissues generally are healthier, while those with fewer methyl groups are likely to lead to health problems. DNA methylation in the pregnant mother is crucial to prevent health problems in children.

Importance of Methylation in the Individual

Consider, for instance, studies done on mice that indicate just how crucial methylation is. Mice, like humans and all other mammals, have a gene called agouti. Methylation in this gene is important, as mice in this study whose agouti genes were completely unmethylated became obese and prone to cancer and diabetes. Their coats were pale yellow.

Meanwhile, genetically identical mice with a methylated agouti gene were of an appropriate body weight, had brown coats (the genetic normal for this variety), and remained healthy, with a low risk of disease. This finding illustrates the mechanism behind one genetic mutation. The mouse DNA is unchanged (except for the removal or addition of methyl groups), but the expression of those genes is radically altered.

Importance of Methylation in Utero

In this same study, pregnant mice with a non-methylated agouti gene (the overweight, yellow mice) were fed a diet rich in methyl. (Some foods crucial in the making of methyl groups are folic acid, B vitamins, and the supplement S-adenosyl methionine.) Though the pregnant mice remained fat and yellow, the majority of baby mice were born with brown coats, did not become overweight, and remained healthy. Thus, the diet of the mother while pregnant can greatly impact the health of her children. This same rule applies to human mothers—it's a lot of the reason behind the sales of prenatal vitamins and the prevalence of prenatal health—the health of a person is attributed not only to his or her individual efforts, but also to the health and nutrition of the mother while pregnant.

Methylation and the Ability to Counteract Detrimental Effects in Utero

One component of plastics, known as bisphenol A (or BPA), has been connected to the development of cancer and other health problems in humans. It's also been shown to reduce agouti methylation in the laboratory. Researchers pitted dietary BPA against a methyl-rich diet in order to determine the extent to which a mother's diet could protect fetal mice from complications.

In this instance, some pregnant mice who were yellow and obese (indicating hypomethylation of the agouti gene) were fed BPA and a normal diet. Another group of the same variety of pregnant, yellow, obese mice was fed BPA as well as a methyl-rich diet. A third group served as a control group.

The results supported the hypothesis that increased methylation can help reduce the risk of health complications due to environmental causes. The mice fed BPA and a regular diet were most likely to have offspring who were yellow and obese. Mice on a regular diet generally gave birth to a mix of healthy, brown mice and obese, yellow mice. Mice who were fed both BPA and a methyl-rich diet were most likely to give birth to slender, healthy, brown mice. Thus, a diet high in methyl not only neutralized the effects of BPA in the maternal diet, it actually counteracted it.

Concerns with Hypo- and Hypermethylation

However, it would be inaccurate to correlate hypermethylation with good health and hypomethylation with disease, as the actual case in humans is much more nuanced.

Some cancers are associated with hypermethylation, though this is usually in regions of DNA that are rich in guanine and cytosine—known as CpG islands. One study of 98 primary cancers (such as (breast, colon, brain, head and neck, testicular, neuroectodermal tumors and acute myeloid leukemia) found that, in general, CpG islands in cancerous tissue are more hypermethylated than the CpG islands in control (non-cancerous) tissue. Specifically, control tissue had a minimum of zero and a maximum of about 4500 hypermethylated CpG islands, while cancerous tissue had an average of 600 - 45,000 hypermethylated CpG islands. Hypermethylation patterns varied with cancer type.

But how does hypermethylation contribute to cancer formation? In particular, when regions of DNA that control transcription are overmethylated, genes that are vital in preventing cancer are silenced, making it possible for cancer to develop and grow.

From this perspective alone, it may seem logical to induce hypomethylation in those with cancer that is associated with hypermethylated DNA. However, while demethylating DNA may initially have an anticancer effect, inducing hypomethylation may actually speed the progression of tumors. This progression is generally sped along because some cancer cells will survive attempted demethylation.

Moreover, in rodent studies, a methyl-deficient diet has been linked to the development of cancer. It is not entirely clear, however, why these low-methyl diets increase cancer risk. Continued studies are needed to completely dissect the relationship between DNA hypo and hypermethylation and the development of cancer.

Of course, hyper- and hypomethylation are inherently subjective terms. More methylation than what? Less than what? In many studies, hypo or hyper refers to having less than or more than the amount of methyl groups in normal tissues. The fact is that "normal" tissues vary in methylation significantly, so plenty of studies compare methylation of cancerous tissues to the noncancerous tissues in the same individual.

It would be easier to discover that hypermethylation is healthy and hypomethylation is not, or vice versa. However, both hypo- and hypermethylated tissues can lead to issues. It depends on individual circumstance when it comes to evaluating cancer risks in people and in other mammals.

Vitamins & Fatty Acids

From childhood, many of us are told to take vitamins, whether it's for general health, energy, bone strength, etc. But many of us don't understand specifically why vitamins are essential and what effects they can have on our genetic expression. Things like choline, Vitamins B, A, D, E, and K are especially important, as is fish oil. Here's why:

Choline & Acetylcholine

This essential nutrient is found in eggs, shrimp, scallops, and cod in very high density. It plays a vital role in methylation in your body, working closing with other B-complex vitamins like B6 and B12. Methylation is a critical biochemical process that is necessary for the proper function of pretty much every system in the body. Methylation takes place billions of times every second to help repair your DNA, control homocysteine, recycle detoxification molecules, maintain good mood, and reduce inflammation. It's also a full support for a neurotransmitter called acetylcholine, whose importance cannot be understated.

In order to maintain focus and attention, your brain needs acetylcholine. In fact, the part of your brain that keeps your heart pumping and your intestines digesting is fueled by acetylcholine. It also plays a huge part in muscle growth, as acetylcholine helps provide a signal that tells your muscles to contract.

B Vitamins

B vitamins have long been hailed as important for energy, but they also have an effect on gene expression on both adult and fetal organisms. Epigenetics and nutrigenomics is a field with relatively limited knowledge, but B vitamins are among the most studied.

One important B vitamin is the water-soluble folate. Dietary folate is responsible for a relatively uncomplicated mechanism of DNA methylation. A methyl group on the folate molecule is used in the synthesis of a unique methyl donor called AdoMet. This donor only supplies methyl groups for DNA methylation reactions. Vitamin B-12 is also a methyl donor for this process. Pregnancies in mothers deficient in folate and B-12 have been shown to lead to obesity in adult offspring, and deficiencies in B vitamins have been linked to several other developmental disorders.

Vitamin A

Vitamin A supplements are frequently sold in drugstores, and vitamin A is one of the better-known vitamins that can affect gene expression. Vitamin A is active in vivo when in the form of retinoic acid. Retinoic acid has been known to reduce effects of inflammatory conditions like psoriasis, acne, and various neoplasias.

Retinoic acid (as well as related substances called retinoids) is able to regulate genes because of its specific binding site. It binds to nuclear receptors in certain cells, and these receptors are ligand-dependent transcription factors. This means that a ligand (the substance binding to them, in this case retinoic acid) is needed to activate transcription. Essentially, vitamin A is necessary to start the DNA transcription process that regulates reduction of inflammation and control of certain conditions.

Vitamin D

Vitamin D is an absolutely essential vitamin, and recent research has shown that it influences over 200 genes. Therefore, a person who has a vitamin D deficiency is much more susceptible to a vast range of conditions.

Vitamin D deficiency is estimated to affect about one billion people. For many, this deficiency is due to inadequate sun exposure. In some cases, though, it's caused by poor diet. In recent research, links between vitamin D deficiency and autoimmune diseases, cancer, and dementia have been uncovered and investigated. Vitamin D is especially important to bone health, as it is vital to proper bone metabolism.

As is the case with most other vitamins, supplementation with vitamin D during pregnancy can increase the likelihood that offspring will be healthier later in life.

Vitamin E

Vitamin E is particularly important to immune response, and in recent years, it has been shown to help counteract some of the effects of aging on the immune system. Supplementing with vitamin E has been shown to significantly impact genes that regulate the cell cycle. It also has a direct effect on T cells—it improves function.

This is helpful in general immune responses, but it is also important for fighting cancer. T-cell therapies have been used to help combat some kinds of cancer, and supplementing with vitamin E can improve the effectiveness of the body's T cells in fighting cancerous or precancerous cells.

Vitamin K

In Japan, vitamin K therapy is used to help patients with osteoporosis, and vitamin K has long been known as a crucial agent in bone metabolism and homeostasis. Research has suggested that vitamin K can increase the activity of osteoblasts, which build bone.

Vitamin K affects genes controlling osteoblast activity indirectly. Vitamin K(2) is able to influence gene expression through a mechanism involving protein kinase A, as well as through a mechanism involving a carboxylase that is dependent on vitamin K. It's possible that future research will reveal more ways that vitamin K signaling pathways can regulate and increase the activity of osteoblasts, which help those who are healing fractures and battling osteoporosis.

Fish oil

Fish oil has long been promoted by nutrition enthusiasts. It contains plenty of omega-3 fatty acids, which can, among other benefits, facilitate the absorption of other supplements (for instance, it aids in the absorption and activity of l-carnitine, a supplement that is found naturally in beef and acts as a mitochondrial catalyst).

However, research has shown that fish oil may have further benefits not known previously. It was known before that fish oil helps fat metabolism in the liver, but newer research shows that it does so by modifying and controlling gene expression of enzymes and transporters that modulate bile acid. In addition, supplementing with fish oil has been shown to modify genes that are related to fat metabolism in both the liver and the small intestine, thus illustrating that fish oil is even more essential than it was already thought to be.

Weight-Loss Supplements: niacin-bound chromium (III), chromium picolinate, and hydroxycitric acid

Weight-loss supplements have been around for what seems like forever. Many are skeptical of them, and for good reason— plenty of weight-loss pills are simply placebos, or they are only pill forms of other dietary elements. You've probably seen green tea pills for sale on the shelves of your pharmacy, or diet pills whose only active ingredient is caffeine. These sorts of pills simply repackage common foods and supplements and add an impressively large price tag. Physicians and dieters are understandably skeptical of this supplement class.

However, certain dietary supplements have been proven to alter gene expression. This does not mean, however, that they are guaranteed to help anyone lose weight. It just means that they have scientific backing—much more so than other diet pills.

However, though some diet pills are ineffective, others may be effective in the wrong way—for instance, the banned substance Ephedra was implicated in several instances of heart damage and even in death. For many, it's wise to wait for research to determine if a given supplement will help in weight loss, and, more importantly, if that drug causes negative effects. Here are some diet pills and supplements and their effects on gene expression.

Niacin-Bound Chromium (III)

Though it is a trace element that can be found in the diet, niacin-bound chromium (NBC) can be sold in supplement form to help those seeking to drop weight and increase lean mass. It is essential for normal metabolism of all essential macronutrients (proteins, carbs, and fat). It promotes a healthy lipid profile, which is essential in everyone.

When taken as a supplement, NBC has been proven to be very safe. The LD50 (the dosage point at which 50 test subjects died) in rats was more than 5000 mg/kg, so a person would have to take unrealistic amounts of the supplement to suffer harm. This particular supplement may modify genetics related to metabolism, but it's extremely unlikely that it would cause adverse effects.

Chromium Picolinate (III)

Chromium picolinate offers an alternative form of chromium. This supplement has been marketed so emphatically that it seems, at first look, to be a miracle supplement. It's been branded as a diet aid with the power to melt fat fast. It's also been hailed as a safe, legal steroid alternative that burns fat while increasing lean gains. The combination of chromium and picolinic acid aids in the absorption of chromium, thus making the process even more effective.

Chromium, while maybe not as miraculous as advertisers claim, is present in foods like poultry, meat, fish, and whole grains. Many people in America are deficient in chromium as a result of the prevalence of processed food. Insufficient chromium generally leads to insulin that is not effective as it could be.

The mechanism of chromium's effectiveness on insulin is unclear, but some hypotheses suggest that it controls the sensitivity of insulin receptors on a genetic level. Claims have been made that chromium boosts serotonin output and reduces appetite that way, though not enough research is available to draw a conclusion.

Hydroxycitric Acid

This is the technical name for what is often marketed as "garcinia cambogia extract." As is the case with many newer supplements, weight loss has been claimed in most of the literature. Since there are very few studies available to date, however, it's impossible to assess its effectiveness over broader populations.

Though it's certainly possible (and likely) that hydroxycitric acid works through regulating gene expression, further research is needed to determine whether or not it does so.

Radiation and Gene Expression

Though perhaps not as well studied as the influence exerted by vitamins on gene expression, research has suggested that different forms of radiation can affect various metabolic processes at the genetic level. This knowledge can be useful for people seeking to modify existing conditions or those who are looking for further connections between environmental influences and genetic expression. Electromagnetic fields (EMF) and radiofrequency radiation (RFR) are two forms of radiation that have been shown to have at least some form of influence on genetic expression.

Electromagnetic fields

Electromagnetic fields can be a powerful force in the process of osteogenesis, or the building of bone. A 2010 study showed that EMFs could benefit osteogenesis in more than one way. When stem cells in bone marrow were exposed to EMFs, cells proliferated 29.6 percent more than cells that were not treated. In addition, on the genetic level, genes treated with EMFs had significantly altered expression of osteogenesis—treated regions of DNA had a 2.7-time increased rate of expression of a key osteogenesis-regulating gene called cbfa1. In addition, EMFs were shown to substantially increase bone mineralization during development, leading to stronger and healthier bones.

While the effect of EMFs on bone cells is relatively well documented, controversy still surrounds its effect on neuroblastoma cells. With more research, the roles of these cells will likely be elucidated.

However, EMFs from mobile phones have been associated with several adverse effects, including sleep disturbances. These are discussed in detail below.

Radiofrequency Radiation

The effects of EMFs on neuroblastoma cells may be unclear, but radiofrequency radiation, also known as RFR, has a much clearer effect on nerve cells. A well-known 1998 report, known as Dr. Henry Lai's Vienna Report on RFR Bioeffects, documents some troubling effects of RFR—a very common form of radiation in our lives—on the brain. What most people don't realize, and what the FCC has done a good job at concealing, is that the most common sources of RFRs are cell phones and cell towers.

RFR can cause DNA damage, and this sort of damage can be especially insidious. It's cumulative, so it doesn't draw the interest that a sudden traumatic brain injury does. In some studies, even a single exposure to RFR damages DNA in the brains of rats. RFR exposure will often cause DNA damage leading to functional changes and to apoptosis (a form of cell death where a cell essentially self-destructs because it is damaged or otherwise different from surrounding cells).

Brain cell damage is especially dangerous because nerve cells do not divide. Most brain cells do not become cancerous, though glial cells can become so after DNA damage.

For those who are especially sensitive to radiation (or who already have cancer and need to avoid radiation as much as possible), listings that rank cell phones in order of emitted radiation are readily available. The increasing availability of headsets and other devices enabling a person to talk on the phone without holding it up at ear level is partially in response to concerns about RFR and neural health.

Other Effects of Radiation

Though EMFs may have been proven to increase bone health, they are responsible for a wide variety of adverse health effects. One such effect is the increase of oxidative stress. This refers to the balance between damaging free radicals and their elimination by antioxidants. Changing this balance can put a person at risk for neurodegenerative diseases and cancer, and it can also increase many of the negative effects of aging.

One study of EMFs surveyed medical students who used mobile phones. It found that students who used a mobile phone for more than two hours each day were much more likely to suffer sleep disturbances. These disturbances contributed to daytime sleepiness, which in turn contributed to decreased cognitive abilities. Studies of people whose occupational hazards exposed them to high levels of EMFs have also indicated that they suffered from more sleep disturbances than the average population.

Sleep disturbances connect to the endocrine system and to general health more than one might think. The body releases a hormone called cortisol in times of stress. For short-term stress, cortisol is effective. Because the body cannot distinguish between short-term and long-term stress, however, it will continue to secrete cortisol in times of prolonged stress. When cortisol is continually secreted, it can lead to weight gain. This is because a stressed body generally (or at least in the wild) needs to hold on to nutrients as much as is possible. In humans, a psychological stress will trigger the same energy-conserving response as a physiological stress.

Additional studies have shown that production of ATP (adenosine triphosphate) is inhibited by exposure to EMF radiation. ATP is crucial for cell activity and general energy. EMFs have been implicated in cases of cancer and other devastating diseases as well. Though more research is needed to develop a conclusive link, EMFs have been linked to the development of Alzheimer's, Parkinson's, Huntington's, and ALS.

Though radiation-blocking technologies have been (and continue to be) developed to combat adverse effects from radiation, one natural remedy—earthing— has been suggested to help level out imbalances.

Many free radicals in the body can accumulate over time, leading to a positive charge. In general, an overall charge that deviates too far from neutral is detrimental to overall health. When a body has too much positive charge, simply standing barefoot on the earth can balance the accumulated charge. This is because the earth has a largely negative charge. Coming into direct contact with earth (no shoes, pavement, etc.) can work to balance out charges and reduce stress. This therapy is also known as "earthing."

The linking of grounding or earthing to reduced positive charge means that, for some, it can reduce the risk of obesity and slow metabolism, as well as reduce the risk of cancer, ALS, and other debilitating diseases. Additionally, studies have indicated that standing barefoot in grass can increase general happiness and well-being. Those who try it have nothing to lose.

Smart Meter Dangers

Certain areas in the U.S. have started using what are known as "smart grids." These grids implement utility meters that transmit information about your home energy use. The info is transmitted in a wireless manner. At some point in time, utilities aim to install these smart meters to each of your home appliances. This will submit your usage data to the previously mentioned smart meter.

Public health might be at risk if this type of technology becomes widespread in the United States. There seems to be a distinct link between rising health complaints in living areas that have smart meters in place. If you visit ElectromagneticHealth.org you can find an in-depth interview about the radio frequencies generated by this new energy-related technology. The high-quality interview features author Blake Levitt, a science writer who wrote *Electromagnetic Fields*. It also features Duncan Campbell, Esq, who provides his insight on the use and development of this new energy-related technology.

Some have noted that EMFs cause difficulty with sleeping and sudden mood swings, both of which are accompanied by headaches.

So, what can you do to guard your health if you must live in a community with smart meters?

You could put up a type of reflective barrier that is designed to protect your meter and your home from radiation. The only issue with this, however, is you must make note of neighboring meters and their precise locations.

If you live in a highly populated area or an apartment community, this may be a pretty big task. You will have to locate and address every single source.

Fortunately, you may request that the meter you have in place only transmit data once per day rather than once per minute. If your house already has a smart meter in place, get in touch with your utility company. You may be able to adjust your transmission rate to once per day. Try to request a time when you are not going to be in your home. Additionally, consider asking your neighbors to do this.

How Exposed Are You To Magnetic Fields?

Since you have running electricity in your home and use a number of appliances that use electricity to function, it is safe to say you're constantly exposed to electric fields. However, the danger of magnetic field exposure is often overlooked, but the ramifications of magnetic field exposure can be just as significant. In order to determine your level of exposure, the magnetic fields must be tested.

Magnetic fields can be generated through a number of different sources. Some of the most common ones are old metal plumbing, nearby power lines, and the motors found on your refrigerator or power meter.

A fairly inexpensive method of testing for magnetic fields is the use of Gauss meter. They are widely available and since you only need to use it once, you can share the costs with friends and family.

Most people don't know this, but using a hair dryer exposes you to magnetic fields. In fact, you get more exposure from this small appliance than from a refrigerator. If you can, limit your use of a hair dryer.

Electric fields can be grounded, but unfortunately, this isn't true for magnetic fields. The only plausible way to ground magnetic fields is to completely encase the culprit using a Faraday cage. Metal provides absolutely no barrier between you and magnetic fields.

There are other appliances in your home that can expose you to magnetic fields, including your laptop and cordless phone base. To avoid exposure, always have a barrier between your lap and your laptop. The thermal and electric fields can be blocked by a pad with reflective material on it. However, it's difficult to fully block magnetic field exposure, so minimize your exposure to these devices.

Charging devices for your computer are never grounded, so use the laptop when it's using battery power and not during the charging routine. The same is true for mobile devices. Women who are pregnant should especially take care not to put themselves in harm's way. Just by switching from a laptop that's plugged in to one that's not, you're decreasing your EMF exposure several hundred times over.

How to Distinguish Between Bad and Good Electromagnetic Fields (EMFs)

Man-Made Harmful EMFs

Since electromagnetic fields, particularly extremely low and very low frequency EMFs, are a much lower strength when compared to other radiation types (such as from X-ray machines or nuclear reactors), researchers used to think they were safe. However, as technology has continued to advance, and electronic devices practically surround us, some researchers have started to suspect that EMFs contribute to subtle attacks on an individual's overall health and immune system function.

Stress-producing electromagnetic fields completely surround us. The fields are generated from the electrical wiring inside our houses and offices as well as from power lines, overhead lights, microwave ovens, video terminals, and hundreds of different kinds of motors generating higher-than-usual Gauss strengths. It is very easy for the human organism's balance to be affected negatively by environmental electromagnetic changes. Unbalanced bodies are much more susceptible to diseases. When living systems interact with EMFs, it can affect the enzymes that relate to cell multiplication and division, growth regulation, and regulation of melatonin (the sleep hormone that the pineal gland metabolism controls).

We are constantly exposed to EMFs—day after day, hour after hour—and this cumulative exposure is a big concern. Larger cumulative exposures of EMFs tend to be generated by ordinary household appliances—cell phones, televisions, computers, kitchen appliances, and electric outlets (especially those directly behind a bed's headboard)—than by power lines, since most people don't live close to power lines. Although EMFs coming from appliances do drop off at about sixteen feet in distance, people tend to be a lot closer to the electromagnetic field source than that. There is hardly any distance at all to cell phones, a couple of feet from televisions, and around eighteen inches from computers.

The first study that established a direct link between cancer and EMFs was conducted at the University of Colorado in 1979. Two epidemiologists, Ed Leeper, PhD, and Nancy Wertheimer, PhD, found that children who were exposed to high-voltage lines when they were young children developed cancer, and especially leukemia, two to three times more frequently than the regular rate.

Dr. Wertheimer's findings were confirmed in 1987 by a large-scale study that the Department of Health for New York State conducted. The study also found that EMFs from high-voltage power lines affected the brain's neurohormones. Since that time, several studies have shown electromagnetic fields being linked to increased incidences in sexual dysfunction, headaches, Alzheimer's disease, high blood pressure, heart disease, and blood disorders, including a 50 percent increase in white blood cell counts.

Man-Made Beneficial EMFs

This refers to frequencies that have been specifically designed and applied in a controlled way. They have more beneficial and natural effects on the body. For home or clinical use, there are devices available for doing pulsed electromagnetic field therapy. According to research, certain pulsed electromagnetic fields with low intensity (gauss) and frequency ranges increase the blood's oxygenation and also improve cell metabolism and circulation. This results in enhanced bone and tissue healing, improved energy levels, reduced inflammation, pain relief, and sound sleep.

Due to these positive effects on the body, using beneficial EMFs on a daily basis helps to support healthy aging processes.

There has been extensive use of EMFs for many medical disciplines and conditions for decades. The results have been shown in both humans and animals.

Man-made beneficial EMFs are identical biologically to frequencies that are created by the body's tissues, bones, organs, and cells. Magnetic fields deliver them to the body, and they are nontoxic and noninvasive.

Food, Breathing, and Sleep

Sleep apnea is an issue that affects many Americans. While you may not have sleep apnea, it's possible that diet could be contributing to an increase in mucus, thus disrupting your breathing and your ability to sleep soundly. Dietary factors can certainly affect gene expression, and they can also disrupt sleep patterns due to physiological processes they set off.

The foods that induce mucus will vary from person to person, but as a general rule, foods that you are allergic to will increase mucus, as will foods that exacerbate acid reflux symptoms.

When you have a history of allergies, it's wise to stay away from foods that you're allergic to. These foods will trigger the release of histamine (as it is released during allergic reactions, even if they are mild) and thereby trigger the production of extra mucus, thicker mucus, or both.

Similarly, when you have acid reflux, your throat can swell and cause mucus to stick. Chances are if you have acid reflux, you know. If you don't have it, some foods that trigger a mucus-forming response are coffee, chocolate, mint, tomatoes, citrus, carbonated beverages, and alcohol. A diet high in fat and the consumption of large meals can also contribute.

As mentioned earlier, sleep stresses can lead to an increase in cortisol, which leads to other adverse effects. These include the altering of metabolic genetics, as the body under stress is programmed to retain nutrients, often in the form of fat.

The popular dieter's adage "food is for fuel" is partially true—food is necessary for powering the body. It's more than that, however. While the body needs calories to sustain life, it also needs a host of micronutrients to maintain proper function. For years, many people considered genetics and environmental factors to be completely separate entities.

This sort of thinking, however, hinders optimal health. When one acknowledges the intersection of diet/environment and genetics, it becomes much easier to understand the body's metabolic processes and, therefore, how to remedy both common and uncommon ailments. Cultivating an understanding of nutrigenomics and epigenetics is crucial to maintaining health. Though it's impossible to absorb all the information in these fields of research, realizing how vitamins and other nutrients interact with your genetics and existing physiology can make it easier to maintain good health and avoid nutritional deficiencies and preventable illnesses.

What This Means for YOU

If you're reading this book, I'm sure you already understand how important your diet and nutrition are. On my blog, I talk at length about foods that help your body and foods that break your body. In one of the articles, "3 Reasons Why You May Not Be Seeing Results at the Gym," I mention how some people consider themselves "non-responders." These individuals are buying into the false notion that they are predisposed to "not respond" to regular exercise and fitness as others do. Clearly, this way of thinking is flawed and only sets you up for failure. The reality is that when you are equipped with the right knowledge, you can actually change your outcomes and achieve your goals.

I've just given you some powerful information as a stepping-stone to taking your health into your own hands. However, I hope it's pretty clear that even if you were to hit the gym five times a week, two times a day, you're not likely to see any results if your nutrition and gene expression are not matching up. I'm going to cover more on this later, but first, I want to share with you something I've previously blogged about.

In the article I spoke about above, I mention Dr. Eric Cobb, creator and co-founder of Z-Health Performance Solutions. He describes the balance so well that I'm going to quote him here:

"What's happening in the big, wide world out there right now is, people are going, 'Well, it must be your genes. It must be you're predestined to not be responsive to exercise.' I personally find that to be a silly concept, a silly idea. So far, nowhere in those studies has anyone mentioned this simple fact that we know to be true… People believe that exercise is so simple that you can't mess it up. That's not true."

Dr. Cobb is 100 percent right about your genes. You are NOT a victim of them. Some people might have "great" genes, which seemingly enables them to achieve awesome results with virtually no effort. In reality, there is often more happening behind the scenes (e.g., hard work in the gym, attention to nutrition, etc.), but contrary to what you're thinking, you don't need different genes to achieve the same results. You need better gene expression.

We have discussed that your thoughts, environment, physical activity, and nutrition all affect blood chemistry, which triggers different gene expression. So, to maximize your health, it makes sense to hit it from all angles. Before blindly throwing darts at the dartboard, though, you need to consider functional testing.

Functional Testing

Up until recently, most gym-goers, personal training clients, and even personal trainers have been using the guess-and-check method to achieve results. They apply a variety of theories and models and observe the outcome. This iterative process generally consists of spinning in circles and never really making any long-term progress. The reason is because guessing—even the most educated guessing—is still guessing. It more often treats symptoms rather than solving root problems.

Functional diagnostic medicine, however, provides an alternative solution. Plus, what better biohack than precision through real lab testing? Functional diagnostic testing allows you to become what Reed Davis, Functional Diagnostic Nutrition founder, calls a "Health Detective." Becoming your own health detective means you regain control and responsibility of your health, and are empowered with data-driven decision-making – a critical component to capturing and improving the bigger picture of your overall health and wellness.

To create new cells our existing cells must divide into two. To do this our cells make copy of our DNA to provide a full set of genetic instructions for the new cell. But sometimes our cells make mistakes during this copying process leading to variations in the genetic sequence at particular locations in the DNA. These mistakes are known as SNPs (pronounced "snips"), or Single Nucleotide Polymorphisms, and testing can shed light to see which of our genetic switches are playing a primary role in our current state of health.

The Role of SNPs in Nutritional Genomics

We are in the era where science is being used to communicate with our bodies to establish their needs. The scientific breakthroughs are being used to determine the complex interaction between foods and genes to unravel new facts about how genetic makeup affect the choice of what the body needs and how it can be customized to meet its demands.

By taking a sample of DNA and passing it through a mass spectrometer, the proteins can be analyzed, and a comprehensive nutritional guide tailored to address these needs. From the research, it has been shown that vitamins, minerals, and other nutrients play a significant role in the manifestation of individual genes in your body. Each of these genes represents a particular function in the body and hence they can be enhanced or suppressed based on their importance to the body. When the genes are at their optimal performance, you will be in a position to reach the ripe old age with minimal disease afflictions.

Genes are regarded as the hereditary factors transferred from the parents to the offspring. They are composed of deoxyribonucleic acid molecules (DNA) which are made up of four nucleic acids; adenine, thymine, cytosine and guanine which are represented by the letters A, T, C, G respectively. The surprising fact is that the DNA of two different individuals is 99.9% identical. You may wonder what makes us different. The remainder 0.1% is considered as the crucial part that differentiates one person from the other. This distinguishing factor is known as the single nucleotide polymorphs (SNPs). The variations in SNPs are used to determine the genetic predispositions of a particular individual. Slight change in the SNP can result in the creation of a different protein molecule and hence the change in the individuals' biochemistry or body metabolism.

Vital SNPs to Analyze

SNP MTHFR-Methylene Tetrahydrofolate Reductase

The Methylene Tetrahydrofolate Reductase gene causes the production of a key enzyme in folate metabolism that handles reducing blood levels of homocysteine. It also plays a significant role in DNA repair and maintenance making new DNA molecules to grow. MTHFR helps in the metabolism of amino acids that make up proteins. Vitamins B12 and B6 are essential for folate metabolism. High levels of homocysteine in the blood can lead to conditions that result in cardiovascular complications.

SNP MTRR- Methionine Synthase Reductase

Methionine Synthase Reductase is an enzyme responsible for maintaining adequate amounts of the vitamin B12, folate and methionine that helps to keep blood levels of homocysteine in check. Low levels of homocysteine are desired for good cardiovascular health. When there is SNP is the MTRR gene of an individual, they are unable to remove adequately the homocysteine that may result in health complications.

SNP SOD- Manganese Superoxide Dismutase

The presence of SNP in the manganese superoxide dismutase makes an individual weak in first line defense against free radicals of superoxide that is harmful to the body. Superoxide dismutase enzyme handles scavenging a process that rids the body of the free radicals. Superoxide is a radical produced abundantly in the cells and usually is the starting point for free radical chain production in the body. Free radical impairs the performance of body cells, accelerates the aging process and also triggers the onset of various types of cancer. According to research, SOD2 is the only enzyme produced in the mitochondria that can scavenge superoxide. SOD3 is mostly found in the placenta, adult heart, the lungs and the pancreas. Increased activity in the body can be an indicator of zinc deficiency to the individual.

SNP VDR – Vitamin D receptor

Vitamin D is critical in promoting the gut absorption of phosphorous and calcium. These two minerals are crucial for the maintenance of proper bone health and reducing cases of osteoporosis among the aging group. The Vitamin D receptor gene accounts for over 75% genetic influence on bone density. The presence of SNP in this gene causes individuals to have reduced bone density than those without the SNP in it. The presence of this gene also influences parathyroid hormone production, young adult growth, blood sugar regulation and healthy cell division.

SNP ApoB- Apolipoprotein B

Apolipoprotein B plays a crucial role in lipid metabolism. Cholesterol, which is a cause of various health afflictions facing humans, is transported in the bloodstream by different lipoproteins; low-density lipoprotein (LDL) and high-density lipoprotein. Alipoproteins are the conjugated proteins that make up the protein part of lipoproteins. The presence of an SNP on ApoB gene causes an increase in ApoB levels which in turn increases total cholesterol levels, triglycerides, LDL cholesterol and impaired glucose tolerance. Suppressing the SNP in this gene can, therefore, cause proper utilization of lipids and hence contributes to better health.

How SNP testing works

Genetic screening involves trial and analysis of the tests to come up with reliable results. It is a simple process that can be performed by taking a blood sample, cheek swabs or any other tissue sampling. One can use any sample that contains one's cell nuclei since the DNA in all the cells are similar. When the DNA is extracted from the sample, it is then amplified, sequenced and put into a readable format for the patient. One can have a single gene, several genes or the entire genome analyzed depending on their needs. Once the results are out, the researcher will then issue a dietary plan tailored to suit your nutritional deficiencies.

Results from SNP testing

One can get an array of information the SNP testing results. Here's what you can attain from SNP testing:

- Identify presence or rare diseases in the body.
- Identify the risk of future diseases associated with genes such as strokes, type II diabetes, Alzheimer's disease, cancers, aneurysms amongst others.
- Identify the current illnesses.
- Identify diseases that you are a carrier and not aware of.

In the next chapter, we will explore the concept of biohacking—shortcuts to desired health outcomes.

Chapter 4

Biohacking

What good is all this information if you don't know how to use it to your benefit? That's a question I'm sure you've already asked yourself. You get it now: our environment and food can affect our genes negatively. But what can you do about it? Well, you can biohack. Biohacking doesn't have a clearly defined description. Semi-officially, it's described as the following:

Biohacking—*the process of fusing tech spirit with biological experimentation in a unique and engaging, non-traditional research setting.*

This concept isn't as scientific as it sounds; many people have conducted experiments with their own bodies and share the information lavishly on the internet. Essentially, biohacking lets you take control of your life and health, providing you a medium where you can see concrete results. Think of biohacking as nutrigenomics put into practice—leveraging science and technology to switch our best genes on and our worst genes off.

If you've ever heard of body cleanses, flushes, detoxes, and fasts, you already understand the fundamental idea behind the concept. When used properly, these types of biohacks are geared towards resetting your system. However, they're typically a short-term solution to reset your current path but can be detrimental when practiced long-term.

So how exactly can you constantly live a life that's on the edge of your capabilities without fasting and detoxing every day?

Utilizing the information you now know about genes and genetic switches, you can start using food to hit those switches that will boost your body with natural energy, brainpower, immunity, and strength. Yes, with simple additions (and subtractions) to your diet, you can start to experience improved digestion, health, strength, energy, and thinking capabilities. That's the power of biohacking!

Tomatoes and Lycopene

I'm sure you've heard that tomatoes are good for you, but do you have any idea why? The body uses antioxidants from fruits and vegetables and turns them into vitamin A. These antioxidants are called carotenoids, and tomatoes have all four major ones: alpha- and beta-carotene, lutein, and lycopene. Together, these combine to provide major health benefits for your body (i.e. hacks for your health, skin, and body).

What I like most about tomatoes is their abundance of lycopene, which is believed to have the highest amounts of antioxidant activity. This high amount of lycopene helps reduce the risk of many different types of cancer—prostate and pancreatic to name two.

Combining tomatoes with other healthy oils and fats, like avocado and pure olive oil, increases your body's ability to absorb the carotenoid phytochemicals up to fifteen times in some cases, according to an Ohio State University study. Moreover, tomatoes are packed with potassium, which most American diets are critically short of.

All these nutrients are great, but how are tomatoes really a biohack? Well, in addition to carotenoids, tomatoes are rich in choline and folate. Also, they have alpha-lipoic acid, which helps the body create energy through glucose, or sugar, conversion. Studies suggest that alpha-lipoic acid helps control blood glucose levels, as well as helps preserve your brain and nerve tissue.

Choline is a great nutrient that helps improve sleep, learning, memory, and even muscle movement. Feeling a bit sluggish? Grab yourself some Celtic Sea Salt. Lower your risk for several types of cancer and help regulate your blood pressure, since the potassium increase to your diet can also increase vasodilation (the expansion of your blood vessels). Your skin is also heavily reliant upon vitamin C, of which tomatoes have a rich supply. This nutrient helps prevent sun damage, as well as other skin damaging exposures, such as pollution and smoke.

If you're prone to depression, enriching your diet with more tomatoes can also help, because they prevent excess homocysteine (a non-protein amino acid) from collecting within the body. Excess homocysteine has been known to prevent blood and other essential nutrients from entering the brain. Therefore, too much negatively affects your body's natural production of serotonin, dopamine, and norepinephrine, which play a significant role in your mood, sleep, and appetite.

Adding tomatoes to your diet doesn't have to be hard. If you eat fast food, please don't rationalize the unhealthy burger because of the iceberg lettuce and wilted tomato slices on your bun. Try dipping cherry tomatoes in hummus or yogurt dip as a snack throughout your day. Learn how to make your marinara sauces from scratch and add canned tomatoes and tomato paste to thicken them up. Your body will thank you for it later!

Tea and Gene Expression

Tea is a favorite for many who dislike coffee or cannot tolerate the acidity of coffee. Epigallocatechin gallate (EGCG) is the active catechin (antioxidant) that gives green tea its incredible healthy reputation. It helps fat cell metabolism and can even clear out abnormal fat accumulation lining the arteries.

One study showed that EGCG can turn on signals to cross a cell membrane and accumulate to the point where gene activity is triggered. In this case, EGCG turned on a pathway called WNT/β- catenin, in which the signal kept fat particles from accumulating in fat cells. That sounds pretty incredible, because science now shows that dieting and losing weight the traditional way raises hormones that stimulate appetite and amplify cravings (making sticking to your diet hard) and lowers certain hormones that suppress your appetite. In other words, when your body has packed on the weight, while it might shed it relatively easily, keeping it off will be a battle.

Green tea gives us an effective way to keep fat cells from accumulating more fat as well as aid in restoring fitness levels to those fatty cells. When EGCG was tested with aortic endothelial cells (artery cells), the results were the same. This means that intense green tea drinkers can enjoy lower risks to fatty plaque formation in these certain types of cells.

Other studies showed that EGCG switched on autophagy genes, too. These types of genes are often described as the house cleaners for cells. When fat begins to pass into cells too fast, energetic abilities are handicapped and eventually are stalled or stopped due to fat accumulation. EGCG helps the cells manage the workload of keeping cells clear of fat. This is how they're able to keep fat from accumulating within the cells.

Excess fat isn't the only thing EGCG ushers out, though. Regular green tea consumption improves and promotes healthy LDL cholesterol levels and functions because of the same approach, ridding the body of excess cholesterol.

Scientists have actually found that several different genes connected to cholesterol metabolism were affected and changed by targeted EGCG treatment. What does that mean for you? Easy: green tea is an effective biohack. If you're attempting to burn off body fat, you definitely want to add this into your diet to help regulate your body's metabolism and excess fat stores.

Coffee

If you're reading this book, chances are you've heard of Bulletproof-style coffee. Perhaps you've even tried it or drink it daily as a part of your quest towards a healthy diet. Or maybe you're a fan of Starbucks and their creamy espressos. Wherever you stand, you should know that coffee has some powerful biohacking properties. But before you go brewing a pot, there are a few things about coffee you should be aware of:

Mycotoxins

During the processing of coffee, there is the potential of extreme exposure to mycotoxins, or in other words, mold growth. In its most simple of definitions, mycotoxins are any substance that has been produced or formed from yeast and fungi.

On my blog, I speak extensively about how mycotoxins are commonly found in our grains and coffee beans. To briefly summarize how they got there, mold toxins come from mold, which grows on weak plant products. And when I say "weak," I mean the immune system of that plant is weak. Why is it weak? Poor farming practices mainly, like planting too many wheat and corn crops, which deplete the soil without replenishing it like green vegetable plants do. When the plants are weak, they emit heat, which bugs have sensory receptors for. Thus, the need for pesticides is increased. Those pesticides seep into the soil and make the plants even more vitamin and mineral deficient. Weak plants are more susceptible to mold, which contaminate coffee even after the roasting process (no, you can't just cook this mold away).

Americans are exposed to this danger through our food sources. I'm talking about our beef (being fed grain), our milk (since dairy cows are fed grain), and our eggs (since chickens are fed grain). These aren't the only ways we're exposed to mycotoxins, though. We're taught to hold on to our food until we see the mold. Truth is, mold is growing long before we can see it, and once you put the spores in your body, they can grow and spread in your body, leading to disastrous results. Coffee is no exception to this rule.

Where Coffee Grows

Coffee comes from a tree, a tropical evergreen from the genus *Coffea*. Most commercial grade coffee comes from just two species grown in this area: *Coffea canephora* (Robustas) and *Coffea arabica* (Arabicas).

It's important to know that the coffee industry production is very labor intensive. Coffee is generally harvested through one of two means: strip picked (by machine) and selectively picked (by hand). There are also two methods for drying out the bean so it can be used for consumption.

The Dry Method

As long as the world has been harvesting the coffee cherry, this is the method that has been used. The method aims to dry the whole cherry, reducing the moisture down to 12.5%. This is done by simply sorting and cleaning the cherries, taking away bad (too ripe, not ripe enough, and damaged) cherries and other particles (dirt, twigs, soil, and leaves).

Once the cherries are ready to be dried, they're laid out in the sun. This sun drying process can take up to a month. So here is where the issue of mold comes into play. Think about your own house if you were to leave something moist and organic out for a month. Sure, it'll dry out alright…but it will also be moldy as heck.

The Wet Method

This method requires some money, as special equipment and large amounts of water are needed for it to be done properly. First, the ripe cherries are cleaned; then they are pulped by a machine that squeezes the cherry to burst the flesh and skin from the bean. What's left is mucilage, the thin slippery outer skin, along with a parchment covering.

The beans are cleaned again to remove any left behind pulp, and then they're placed in large tanks. In those tanks filled with water, the mucilage is eaten away by natural enzymes and then washed away again. This is a type of fermentation (spoiling) that removes the outer layer and is actually quite quick, taking a mere 24 to 36 hours. At this point, the coffee bean is at about 57% moisture.

That's way too high, so the remaining parchment coffee bean is usually dried with a combination of the sun and a mechanical dryer. Using this method, sun drying will only take about eight to ten days.

The wet method is preferable as it yields little to no mycotoxins. Fair-trade, wet-processed coffee is selectively picked, meticulously dried, and roasted under ideal conditions to yield the cleanest coffee. This type of coffee is likely to have the lowest mycotoxin content possible. Typically, very expensive craft coffees, Kona Coffee, and some local organic coffees will use this method. When in doubt, ask the coffee provider which method they use.

Bulletproof-Style Coffee

How well coffee boosts your system depends solely on where your coffee has been grown and, most importantly, how it is dried. Cheap coffee usually comes from the dry method or a mix of the two. Sure, the caffeine will give you a little physical energy boost, but you're likely to still feel sluggish, both physically and mentally.

Perhaps you shake and have the jitters or experience the terrible crashes associated with tremendous caffeine spikes. If you would like coffee to really boost your body, you should definitely consider blending the following ingredients into your next cup of coffee to create Bulletproof-style coffee:

- 2 Tbsp Kerrygold unsalted grass-fed butter or raw cream
- Pinch of Celtic or Himalayan sea salt
- 2 cups of organic, fair-trade coffee
- Stevia (non-GMO) to taste

While it may seem odd to add more fat to your daily diet, the truth is that most people aren't consuming enough healthy saturated fats. Again, this is something I would verify by getting your labs done with a functional medicine doctor (Essential & Metabolic Fatty Acids Analysis). However, if you'd like to try this recipe, start with small amounts of butter before working your way up to more. I would also suggest taking digestive enzymes with this to help break these fatty acids down until your gut has adapted. Digestive proteolytic enzymes such as bromeline and papain, and betaine HCL can be helpful when you're not able to get enough natural enzymes from food.

As we discussed before, your DNA stores the code for all of your body's proteins and enzymes. Genetic disease is commonly a result of your DNA improperly or inadequately producing proteins and enzymes. Bacteria, fungi, yeast, and viruses are protected by proteins that our immune system must attack to keep us healthy. Additionally, food allergens are mostly proteins and cancer cells are protected by proteins. So supplementing with proteolytic enzymes can not only aid digestion but also the digestion and destruction of the protein shield of every pathogen, allergen, and rogue cells.

Personally, I drink a perfect cup of Bulletproof-style coffee almost every morning. Keeps me alert and on my toes.

Now, it's not just this style of coffee that can have a powerful effect on your genes but the coffee itself has been shown in studies to positively influence epigenetics. Let's explore the role of coffee itself in nutrigenomics.

As one of the world's most popular drinks, coffee has received much notoriety on its seemingly contradictory health benefits and risks. Whether or not coffee is actually good for you has been the subject of debate for decades. So, with all of the conflicting information floating out there, how do you know if it's actually good for *you*?

First, let's look at some interesting coffee stats:

- Coffee houses in 17th century England were called penny universities since you could buy a cup of coffee for a penny and have intellectually stimulating conversations as a result
- Today, we drink 730 billion cups of coffee worldwide
- A typical 150 mL cup of coffee contains 40-180 mg of caffeine
- People in the US drink on average two cups of coffee per day, while Europeans drink four

Worldwide, coffee has been known to promote wakefulness, enhance mood and cognition, and provide a stimulant effect. However, the scientific basis for coffee's health benefits seems to be full of contradictions. Tolerance to the effects of coffee seems to build quickly for some and actually very slowly for others. It also seems that at low doses, the psychological effects of coffee include alertness and enhanced cognition, but some people feel anxious, nauseous, and jittery.

It appears that what coffee may provide for some it does not provide for others. For some, coffee can help reduce the risk for brain stroke, Parkinson's disease, liver disease, and type 2 diabetes. For others, however, coffee seems to actually *increase* their risk for pre-diabetes. Some people develop high blood pressure from coffee whereas others don't. Some benefit from its heart-protective benefits, and others don't. Some experience a reduced risk of cancer and tumors, while for others it may seem to do nothing at all.

So are the scientific studies all wrong, or does each us respond differently to coffee? I think you know where I'm going with this. Scientists have concluded that some would benefit from reducing their intake of coffee while others would benefit from increasing it. So it should be apparent that your genes impact your response to coffee. But the question is, how?

Fortunately, Harvard scientists have led the largest genome-wide association study on coffee consumption to date. The scientists looked at the entire genetic code of 129,488 European and African American coffee drinkers. Some of these coffee drinkers were infrequent drinkers and some drank coffee frequently. From the study, they were able to identify individual genetic differences in single nucleotide polymorphisms (SNPs) which were associated with their coffee drinking behavior.

From analyzing the SNPs they found how your genes influence whether coffee is good for you or not. What's more is that the scientists also discovered six new gene variants linked to frequent coffee drinking (POR, ABCG2, GCKR, MLXIPL, BDNF, and SLC6A4) and re-confirmed two other variants found in former research (AHR and CYP1A2). So they found eight coffee-related gene variants in total. Geneticists call this a "complex trait" because it requires the interplay of many genes.

From these eight genetic variants, scientists found that:

- Genes GCKR and MLXIPL, which are involved in sugar and fat metabolism, are associated with the metabolic and neurological effects of caffeine. People with these gene variants enjoy the stimulant effects of coffee more than others.

- Two areas of DNA near the genes BDNF and SLC6A4 participate in creating a "reward" effect in your brain when drinking coffee, which increases the motivation to drink coffee. BDNF specifically controls the activity of serotonin, glutamate, dopamine, and other neurotransmitters in the brain that influence memory, learning, and mood. Some people who have a mutation on the BDNF gene experience less of the reward effects of coffee and thus a decreased desire to drink it.

- Genes POR and ABCG2 are involved in metabolizing caffeine by encoding specific proteins to break caffeine down. Frequent coffee drinkers with a tolerance for caffeine have increased expression of these two genes. This allows them to metabolize coffee better and more quickly than infrequent coffee drinkers.

- The gene AHR plays a role in the brain pathways that stimulate coffee drinking.

- CYP1A2 stimulates the breakdown of coffee and caffeine levels in the blood stream. People with this gene variant can detoxify the effects of coffee faster and have a much higher tolerance to it.

So, you can see the essence of what studies like this tell us—your genetic expression influences your behavior and experience with foods such as coffee drinking. I'm sure you've also witnessed the phenomena of those that can metabolize coffee quickly vs. those that can't (i.e. fast vs. slow caffeine metabolizers). The enzyme in the liver primarily responsible for this is cytochrome P450 1A2 (CYP1A2). One study from 2006 found that those with variant CYP1A2*1A metabolize caffeine quickly, while those with CYP1A2*1F metabolize caffeine much more slowly. This explains why fast metabolizers generally need more coffee to feel the same stimulating effects.

The interesting thing is that the health benefits of coffee for fast vs. slow caffeine metabolizers differ greatly. Slow caffeine metabolizers experience a significantly increased risk of non-fatal heart attack from only 2-3 cups of daily coffee consumption, whereas fast caffeine metabolizers actually experience a reduced risk of heart attack from the same daily consumption. What this ultimately means is that slow caffeine metabolizers should still be able to drink 1-2 cups of coffee per day to experience the brain health benefits without the adverse effects. Another interesting fact is that coffee, not caffeine, is associated with lower risks of type 2 diabetes and cancer. If you decide to choose decaf coffee as an option, aim for one with a healthier decaffeination process such as those made from water processed or CO_2 extracted coffee beans.

Before ordering a genetic test to see what type of coffee metabolizer you are, look at your coffee drinking habits as they are naturally modulated by your genetic expression. If you do decide to get genetic testing done, be mindful of that fact that consumer tests like 23andMe don't provide your entire genome sequence. They, instead, selectively pick genes and variants rather than analyzing the entire DNA sequence. Specifically, make sure to check if the test includes the gene variants I've discussed here.

So are you drinking too much or too little? Well, the European Food Safety Authority considers 400 mg of caffeine per day to be safe for healthy adults. Your key takeaway here isn't that you should become a caffeine junky. The main point here is that the paradoxical controversy surrounding coffee's health benefits are a clear sign that it's not so much about coffee as it is about YOU. Your individual genetic makeup and genetic expression is the best indicator of whether coffee will do great things for your health or have disastrous consequence

Chapter 5

Fat Burning and Muscle Gain

We're finally ready to talk about fat loss and muscle growth in light of nutrigenomics and the boatload of information you've just downloaded. It's not uncommon for people to think that if they just drink a couple of protein shakes a day and make their muscles burn at the gym, then they're on the right path. I cannot stress to you enough how many people unknowingly cause themselves more damage (and/or no results) simply because they lack the requisite knowledge. If you're serious about getting to the root of what keeps you unfit and unhealthy, then you're in the right place.

We're going to discuss how your body functions daily. We will explore how your body generates energy and how stress, both psychological and physiological, affects your body. We're also going to discuss how muscle and fat play a part in your fitness levels. All of this information will play a huge role in using nutrigenomics to attain the health and body you have always desired.

How the Body Functions Daily

The daily functions of your body can be broken down into a series of functions and systems. Many of them operate without us even having to think about them. The most common of the automatic systems are those regulating our beating heart and breathing.

The following systems make up the daily functions of our body:

Circulatory System—Moves blood, oxygen, nutrients, hormones, and carbon dioxide around the body.

Digestive System—Is made up of organs that help break down food so that its nutrients can be absorbed and its remains excreted.

Endocrine System—This system secretes the hormones regulating metabolism, sexual function, and growth into the bloodstream.

Immune System—Your body's internal defense system against bacteria, toxic pathogens, and viruses.

Lymphatic System—This system involves lymph nodes, ducts, and vessels and helps the immune system in the body's internal defense.

Nervous System—Involving both involuntary (breathing and heart rate) and voluntary (conscious movements and breathing) functions, this system contains the nerves that allow us to touch, taste, feel, hear, and see. This system not only governs all other systems, but also controls our thought processes and emotions.

Muscular System—Contains the regulatory power of the 650 muscles that allow second-by-second movement, blood flow, and other bodily functions such as digestion, heart regulation, and breathing.

Reproductive System—Just what it says. Wanna make babies, create new life, and have fun at the same time? Tip your hat towards this system. Best. Thing. Ever. Moving on…

Skeletal System—Our muscles, organs, skin, and blood would be nothing without the 206 bones erecting it along with cartilage, ligaments, and tendons. It also stores calcium and helps in the production of blood cells.

Respiratory System—Our brain wouldn't survive without the ability to breathe in oxygen and exhale the byproduct of carbon dioxide.

Urinary System—Digesting food and carrying out bodily functions creates a waste called urea, known to us as urine. We have to get it out somehow, and the urinary system is how we do that.

Integumentary System—Our skin—and it does more than just cover our innards. First defense against the outside, it also helps regulate internal body temperature and excrete waste through perspiration.

I wanted to give you a complete list of the body's systems so that you'd know just what systems rely upon protein synthesis and nutrients for energy—all of them. When your body is off kilter, you can expect the above systems to be affected. The muscular system is probably the most known system to be affected by a surplus or deficiency of essential nutrients and proteins in the body, which we'll talk about next, but know that all systems are affected by your nutrition.

How Muscle Is Made

In my book, *Nutriscribe*, I devote a whole chapter to how energy is created and released during workout sessions and weight training. What I didn't mention in that book, though, is that muscle growth happens when muscle protein synthesis occurs at a rate greater than muscle protein breakdown. Protein breakdown is bad; protein synthesis is good.

In addition to this rate of growth vs. break down, after a good workout, your body sets to work repairing and replacing any damaged muscle fibers. This is done through a process that fuses fibers together in order to form new strands of muscle protein, or myofibrils. The myofibril that is fused during this process creates thickness and growth. In other words, this is how you get fit, toned, and just plain good looking.

How Muscles Grow

If you are a guy who hits the gym and trains with weights, then the chances are you are looking to gain some muscle, on top of losing some fat. This is why I want to shed light on the mechanisms of how muscles actually grow. Plus, I want to discuss why many women won't actually pack on a bunch of muscle while training with weights. I want to point out that there are many types of muscles, including heart muscle, but we will be discussing skeletal muscles. These types of muscles are made up of myofibrils, as well as sarcomeres, which form muscle fibers, and they are actually the basic units of muscle contraction.

As for how many skeletal muscles are in the body, there are hundreds. As a matter of fact, there are 650 of them, and when they receive signals from motor neurons, they contract. These motor neurons are important, as they let your muscles know that they should contract. The better you are at having such signals tell your muscles what to do (contract), then the stronger you can get. This is important to remember.

Many power lifters can lift a bunch of heavy weight, but they may not look that muscular. They have the ability to activate the motor neurons and, as a result, they are able to contract their muscles in a better manner. This is why some power lifters are smaller than bodybuilders, but are stronger than them. Let's not forget to mention that motor unit recruitment plays a role in explaining why some movements become easier to do (after practice). After this initial period is when muscle growth tends to take place, and this is because the muscles can usually be activated more easily.

1. Muscle Growth: The Physiology Behind It—After you have completed a workout, your muscle fibers are replaced (the damaged ones) or repaired via a process that involves muscles fibers being fused together in order to form brand new protein strands, or brand new myofibrils. These new strands that have been repaired are thicker and they increase in number, which in turns create muscle growth, or muscle hypertrophy. Something you should remember is that muscle growth happens when the rate of protein synthesis is greater than the rate in which protein in the muscle breaks down. This actually happens while you are resting, and not when you are hitting the weights.

You may be wondering how you exactly add more muscle to the muscle cells, and this is where satellite cells come into play. Long story short, these satellite cells can become activated, and when they are, they serve as stem cells for your muscles, and also play a role in adding more nuclei to the cells. This eventually leads to the growth of myofibrils. These cells may be what leads to people being able to grow extremely massive muscles, as well as what causes people with a lack thereof to be classified as hard-gainers.

It's worth mentioning that there have been a number of studies that have shown that the people who were extreme responders to muscle growth had around 20% activation of satellite cells. Those who were considered to be modest responders had a little less than that. Some of the non-responders had no growth at all, as well as 0% activation of satellite cells. So what does this actually mean? It means that the more these cells can be activated, the more you could grow. So how do you activate these cells when you want to gain more muscle?

2. The 3 Mechanisms That Allow Muscles to Grow—You need to put more stress on muscles if you want them to grow, and you need to do this often. As a matter of fact, stress is one of the major factors involved with muscle growth, along with the force of homeostasis. This causes three main mechanisms that lead to muscle growth, which will be discussed below.

The first mechanism is muscle tension, which means you need to apply a whole bunch of stress that your body and muscles are not adapted too. One way you can do this is by lifting heavier weights and progressing with it as time goes on. The chemistry of your muscles will eventually be changed up and this means satellite cell activation could take place and you could pack on some more muscle. Let's not forget to mention that tension can affect the connection between motor units and muscle cells, which is possibly why some people may not be big, but are extremely strong.

The second mechanism is muscle damage, which you may experience when you are sore after training, or when you feel localized soreness, which is also known as localized muscle damage. This is a result of inflammatory molecules and immune system cells being released, and satellite cells jumping into action. However, it's worth pointing out that just because you don't feel sore doesn't mean that this doesn't happen. Other mechanisms can attenuate the soreness that you might otherwise feel.

The third mechanism is metabolic stress, which is usually felt in the form of a 'burn' or when you have a 'pump' after you have trained. Bodybuilders were questioned about how a pump caused their muscles to be bigger, and eventually an investigation was launched. The investigation revealed that these bodybuilders were definitely onto something.

You see, cells that are around your muscles end up becoming swelled due to metabolic stress, and this actually helps contribute to the growth of muscle. Muscle glycogen also plays a role in making muscles pumped up. In other words, this type of muscle growth is one of the ways people can look bigger without getting stronger. The next thing we will discuss is how hormones can affect growing muscles.

3. Hormones And How They Affect Muscle Growth— Hormones affect muscle growth, as they can regulate satellite cell activity. Also, testosterone and MGF (mechano-growth factor) play a huge role in muscle growth. Testosterone is one of the major hormones that people think about when it comes to training with weights, and one reason is because it increases protein synthesis, as well as activates satellite cells. It even stimulates anabolic hormones. Strength training also helps releases more of this hormone into the body. Long story short, when more testosterone is released into the body, there is a greater potential for muscle growth and a stimulation of growth hormone.

As for the IGF, or insulin growth factor, it regulates muscle growth, and it does this by enhancing protein synthesis. Not only that, but it stimulates the uptake of amino acids. Once again, it also activates satellite cells, which helps increase muscle growth.

4. Rest Is Important For Muscle Growth—It is important for you to get proper rest consistently if you want your muscles to grow because even a slight deficiency of rest over time forces your body into a destructive state metabolically. While gender, genetics, and age will all help determine your muscle growth— for example, men have more testosterone than women, and this allows men to build stronger and larger muscles—rest is universally valuable. Regardless if you are a man or woman, you need to get adequate rest in order for your muscles to grow.

Sleep For Muscle Growth

Enough sleep is as important in body building as eating well and training regularly. The first step to gaining muscle mass is by eating nutritious and well-balanced meals, followed by spending some time training and lifting weights. Although proper nutrition and body exercise are mandatory for bodybuilding and muscle growth, enough sleep and rest does play a big role in this. Sleep is one aspect most people do not take into consideration in bodybuilding.

How Sleep Affects Muscle Growth

Every time you work out, your muscles degenerate and tear at the cellular level. The degenerated and injured cells need time to heal for the muscle tissue to strengthen. The only way these cells can be repaired is by eating well-balanced and highly nutritional meals and by getting enough sleep. Taking some time to relax also helps rejuvenate muscle cells.

The body also enters a heightened anabolic state when one is asleep. It is at this time that body tissues and cells are repaired. It is also during this time that the body starts regenerating larger cell molecules meant for increasing muscle mass and toning. Researchers also believe that our immune systems improve when we get enough sleep, and so do the muscular and nervous systems.

How Much Sleep Is Enough?

The body conducts protein metabolism more efficiently when one is asleep as compared to while awake. This makes sleep crucial for anyone looking for a way to build muscle mass or gain weight. Sleep is also critical for muscle repair as it encourages faster recovery, especially of injured tissues. Sleep is also vital for strength training as it helps you train much better and take on even heavier tasks the next day. Doctors and researchers therefore recommend at least eight to ten hours of sleep daily.

It is however advisable not to oversleep, as this will reset the body's sleep schedule, making it hard for you to find sleep the next day.

Muscle Growth and Sleep: The Effects

The body requires enough sleep cycles for full cell tissue repair and recovery. The body also produces high amounts of melatonin and testosterone hormones while one is asleep. This is mostly true in men who produce high amounts of testosterone while they are asleep. These hormones are vital for cell regeneration and reproduction and hence improve muscle growth. Anyone who doesn't get enough sleep isn't capable of producing enough of these hormones, hence muscle development and growth is retarded.

Muscle Tissue Production

For the body to generate more muscle mass, it has to synthesize more proteins faster than it is burning the same. Synthesized proteins are vital as they not only help repair cells and tissues, but also promote muscle growth. There is a greater chance that the body will break down already synthesized proteins when one is asleep. This is the reason why it's advisable to eat plenty of proteins before going to bed and to have a heavy breakfast as well. It is during sleep that the body will synthesize and use these proteins for muscle growth and development.

Inhibit Protein Breakdown with Amino Acids

Raising amino acid levels in the body is the best way of preventing breakdown of proteins. The best way to do this is by taking whey protein isolate before bed and getting enough sleep. Whey proteins help increase amino acid presence in the body, which means the body will have to use that up before turning to already synthesized proteins. Casein protein is another good alternative for whey proteins, as it lasts much longer.

Sleep and Cortisol Production

Cortisol is a hormone you wouldn't want in your body especially when in a body-building venture. Cortisol is mostly produced by lack of sleep, stress, and lack of enough nutrients to support muscle growth. Cortisol is also the one hormone that inhibits testosterone production, making it hard for muscle growth to occur. Getting enough sleep however helps inhibit cortisol production and promotes testosterone production. This is evidence enough that sleep is mandatory for muscle growth.

5. Why Rapid Growth Of Muscles Is Unlikely—The majority of people find that muscle hypertrophy takers quite a bit of time and is slow, which means it could take weeks or even months for them to see any changes to their physique. Not only that, but people have varying hormonal output, genetics, and types of fibers, and all of these things can play a role in how much muscle growth a person can see and how fast it takes them to pack on muscle. However, when you do see results, chances are you will become highly motivated, which can play a huge role in gaining muscle over a period of time.

Long story short, you need to force your muscles to adapt, and you do this by providing it with more stress than before. You do this by lifting heavier, for instance, and progressing your workout routine. Also, don't forget to rest because this is important, and you need to eat properly in order for your muscles to grow.

Satellite Cells

Myosatellite cells are contained in mature muscle. When they're activated, they help add more live muscle cells and directly affect the growth rate of myofibrils. Turning these myosatellite cells on is believed to be what allows some individuals to grow muscles more effectively while others may struggle to remain at a modest level of muscle retention.

Within the past five years, studies have revealed that those gaining 58% in myofibrils (muscle fibers) after an exercise bout had an astounding 23% activation among their satellite cells.

Can you imagine that? Just 23% activation yielded an incredible 58% increase in muscle cell growth!

How Fat Is Burned

This section isn't about the top 21 ways to shed body fat fast. I don't believe in those gimmicks, and you shouldn't either. Instead, I'm going to approach fat and mass weight loss from the physiological standpoint.

When you shed weight, it doesn't melt into thin air. Instead, it changes form, just like water and ice.

Normally, our body processes carbohydrates to extract glucose and sugar. The liver stores the glucose, releasing it into the bloodstream as needed. Once the glucose has been used, the body starts to burn fat. Creating energy by burning fat is a metabolic state known as ketosis.

Ketosis

This is the state that many fitness competitors want to achieve because they believe it will trick their body into burning more fat. Sure, why workout when your body can just burn your fat for energy? Sounds like a win-win situation, right? It can be beneficial if it's only for a short period of time. However, long periods of ketosis are extremely hard on your kidneys and other organs.

If used appropriately, as I'll show you in a second, ketosis can yield some pretty amazing results for fat metabolism. Below is a strategy to biohack your way safely into and out of ketosis, to shed fat fast:

Carbohydrate Cycling Example 1:

Menu 1
150 g protein
33 g carbs
30 g fat

Menu 2
150 g protein
95 g carbs
30 g fat

Menu 3
150 g protein
125 g carbs
45 g fat

Menu 4
150 g protein
33 g carbs
85 g fat

*These recommendations are based on a 125 lb female.

Sample Week:

- Monday—Menu 1
- Tuesday—Menu 1
- Wednesday—Menu 4
- Thursday—Menu 2
- Friday—Menu 1
- Saturday—Menu 1
- Sunday—Menu 3

Please be aware that this strategy is not for everyone and should only be considered once all of your fundamental nutrition requirements have been met (i.e., enough protein, green vegetables, good fats, water intake, eating to 80% full, etc.). For more about this, check out my book *Nutriscribe*.

Scientifically, here's why this works: Hormones that keep watch on our blood sugar levels activate an enzyme called lipase (which specifically breaks down fat cells) located within the blood vessels of fatty tissue. Lipase, in turn, ignites surrounding fat cells to release triglycerides and glycerol.

Triglycerides are what make fatty cells fat. When lipase is released, they get the signal to leave the fat cells and break down into their separate parts. Once separated, they enter into the bloodstream where the glycerol is snatched up by the liver to process for energy while the rest of the fatty acids move to nearby muscles that will use them for energy, too. The process of breaking lipase down for usable energy is called lipolysis.

Lipolysis

This action creates the fabulous ATP that makes sweating it out at the gym possible. When fatty acids and glycerol enter into cells from the bloodstream, they're taken in by mitochondria, which are known as the powerhouses of the cells in muscles and the liver. These broken-down components are shifted to create heat, carbon dioxide, water, and a weight trainer's best friend, adenosine triphosphate (ATP). The water is excreted as sweat, and we exhale the carbon dioxide.

You're Not a Victim of Your Genes

When it comes to losing weight, I really feel that many fitness sites just have it wrong. They produce a list of how to slash your calories, curtail your carbs, and sweat it out for at least 30 minutes a day to see results. Instead, what ends up happening is that some people lose weight while the others end up feeling like exercise must just not "be for them."

The truth is that most "diets," if not all, make you drop your water weight first, muscle second, and then perhaps a little fat. When we diet alone (especially crash diet), we lose up to 20% to 40% muscle. This muscle loss causes our body to store up any fat left hanging around by slowing down our metabolism.

Since researchers have discovered the role that gene expression or suppression plays in regulating fat loss and muscle growth, they've realized that the body does resist shedding pounds.

Researchers from Sweden's Department of Clinical Sciences Malmo discovered seven key genes that are expressed within adipose (fat) tissue that change with both weight maintenance and weight loss. This finding helps to bring science a step closer to better understanding how the human body regulates and responds to fat loss.

The randomized controlled trial found that the genes that the adipose tissue expressed undergo changes when an obese individual loses weight and keeps it off. The authors reported that for most people it was a difficult yet important task for them to maintain a level of reduced weight in order to fully benefit from losing weight.

Twelve obese adults were placed on a low calorie diet for a period of three months. Once the subjects had lost 10 percent of their total body weight, they next went on a six month weight maintenance program. The researchers took blood and adipose samples at baseline, right after weight loss and then after the weight maintenance period.

The researchers reported that participants lost an average of nearly 19 percent of their body weight. In addition, immediately after the weight loss phase, there were improvements in blood triglycerides and insulin sensitivity. After weight loss was sustained, there were also improvements in HDL ("good" cholesterol).

Gene Expression

The researchers reported that 2,163 genes in total were affected during the weight loss period and during weight maintenance there were modifications to 1,877 different genes. Two of the genes that were expressed the most strongly, ABCG1 and CETP, were most likely responsible for the HDL improvements that were found following sustained weight loss. When there is a high level of HDL it provides the body with a higher capacity for clearing cholesterol out of the tissues and then returning it to the liver so that it can be excreted or recycled. Both of the genes code for enzymes which promote the transfer of cholesterol to HDL-mobilizing cholesterol in such a way that losing weight might effectively boost the health of the heart and overall function of the body.

A majority of dieters have discovered that their bodies resist weight change. Research findings have shown that the expression of CIDEA, the weight-guarding gene, is higher in subjects who are trying to maintain weight loss. Blocking the expression of CIDEA in mice prevented weight gain even when they were over fed. The increased CIDEA expression in subjects attempting to prolong their weight loss efforts exemplifies how rapid weight loss sabotages health by sinking metabolic rate.

An individual who carries too much weight for their height and body type also carries too much stress as well. Many problems that are associated with obesity are due to the fact that the body is attempting to cope with it. Two genes were focused on by the researchers: TNMD and MMP9. As a result of weight maintenance and weight loss, they were down-regulated. TNMD and MMP9 are genes that might be responsible for adapting to conditions such as metabolic syndrome and obesity.

MMP9 codes for the metallopeptidase cell structure, which is frequently referred to as the metallopeptidase matrix. As author Amanda Jensen from Evolving Health writes, it is like the scaffolding of a building that can be degraded, modified or moved. The metallopeptidases are the cells' contractors. When there are fewer MMPs there are less cells that are built up and broken down. The overall result is possibly smaller but more fat cells.

TNMD codes for tenomodulin, which is a protein. It is the modulator or contractor of blood vessels. In obese individuals TNMD is higher. It has been linked to poor control of blood sugar and fat mass. The authors of the study reported that low amounts of matrix metallopeptidase 9 and tenomodulin or other related proteins might be important for weight loss beneficial effects.

Weight Maintenance

It was once thought that adipose tissue was an added layer of insulation and dormant energy store receptacle. However, it is actually a metabolically active organ. Fat cells really do perform work and function. The researchers report that they contain genes affecting metabolism, hormonal balance and immune response- which are all involved in the creation of setting a point for weight.

Losing weight is not easy to do, particularly when your body views fat as a form of security. For many it can be an uphill battle trying to lose weight, plus with each extreme weight loss effort, where weight is lost and rebounded, it makes it harder and harder for the individual to lose weight. When weight is lost, the body starts to fight for its stores of fat; metabolic rate shifts, satiety is impaired and hormones change. According to researchers, this resilience is mostly due to genes being expressed.

The researchers recommend that the focus of future research on weight loss beneficial effects should be on assessing the long-term effects following the weight stability period. The results provide interesting insights into fat physiology and its genetic adaptations. Anybody can lose weight. However, correctly sustaining it is the battle that has the true benefits according to the researchers.

Supplements: Why Take Supplements?

Before we dive in to an extensive collection of research on some wildly alternative supplement options, I want to take a moment and discuss why you should even consider adding supplements to your daily diet regimen. At one point, I was just like any other American. I truly believed that I could get my vitamins from my regular diet and that I didn't need any type of additional supplement. If you conduct your own research on the need for supplements, you'll find very few sites and places advocating the need for such an addition to your diet. Most dietary sites tend to take a very cautious approach to supplements, stating that it's important to decide if you even need them or not.

I could write an entire article on the needs and benefits of taking supplements, but for the purposes of this book, I'll keep it simple and give you a few common reasons that you may or may not already be aware of.

First things first: you need to understand that a regular American diet isn't all that nutritious, even if you only eat organic. Sure, plants can be deemed certified organic, but improper farming techniques and practices, such as repeatedly growing crops on the same plot of land, can cause the soil to lose vitally important nutrients needed to both sustain crops to harvest and to support human health.

Today, many farmers use nutrient-boosting fertilizers that help plants survive until harvest time, but don't necessarily support quality human health when eaten. A UK study confirmed this finding, showing that copper levels had dropped 90% in dairy, 76% in vegetables, and 55% in meat. What does all this mean? That the food you eat, even if it's organic, simply may not contain the vitamins your body needs.

The other side to simply relying on your diet is the fact that even if your food is incredibly rich and nutritious, your body may not be absorbing all the vitamins and minerals that food contains. Grains and legumes have been known to cause intestinal damage that can affect your ability to absorb the nutrients in your food. Even if you were to stop eating foods that have been proven to cause damage to your gut, the existing injuries could still prevent future absorption.

This sounds like a bunch of downer information. I'm telling you this because you need to know the facts. Your diet and exercise alone might not be enough. This doesn't mean that you're not doing a good job of taking care of yourself; it just means that your body needs a little help, a boost, if you will. This is where supplements can come in to save the day.

Hold on, though—don't rush out the door to the grocery store down the street with the lame buy-one-get-one-free ad. I wouldn't trust commercial grade supplements simply because they're not likely to be produced with the same care that other natural, more organic compounds will be. I had a friend self-diagnose himself with insomnia. He tried everything and still couldn't get himself to sleep at night, no matter how tired, exhausted, or fatigued he was. His solution? He tried the standard melatonin pills available from a local grocer. Don't be surprised—he didn't see any results until he was seen a doctor prescribed medical grade melatonin. Even that prescription stopped helping after a while, and I'm talking a period less than three months. After more research, he finally found some relief with traditional medicine used in other countries but not necessarily in America. You'll find out more about that in our supplements section a little later on. First, let's keep talking store brand supplement pills.

It's not uncommon for many people to raid the dietary sections of grocery stores and feel like they've done the best they can because they started taking supplements. Remember, if you don't see any results, you're wasting your time and your money. Take a look at the following supplements I've researched for you. If any one of them catches your eye, conduct some further research and collect all the information you feel you need before making a decision. All or most of the following supplements are available through Superman Herbs online. I recommend them because their products are high in quality and sometimes even taste (although taste simply can't be helped with some herbs).

Pine Pollen

Yes, I'm talking about the annoying yellow coat of dust on your cars and windows each spring. Thanks to incredible research by Stephan Harrod Buhner, author of *Pine Pollen: Ancient Medicine for a Modern World*, we can now begin to understand in the West why the Chinese have used this substance in their traditional medicine for so many years.

This type of supplement has incredible benefits for both men and women for its unprecedented testosterone boosting capabilities (for an all-natural herb). And unlike artificial testosterone boosters or synthetic derivatives of testosterone, this herb keeps your estrogen and testosterone in better balance, which means you avoid the common side effects like breast development in men and over masculinization in women. The number of human androgens (natural hormones often found in men) it contains boost testosterone levels in men within minutes. Sure, we're talking increased libido, but we're also talking more restorative sleep, superhuman strength, and boundless energy to do the things you love.

Pine pollen also contains natural prostate regulators called gibberellins, which helps maintain a healthy prostate size. And this is just the beginning! Pine pollen has been used in traditional Chinese medicine for thousands of years, so they know the benefits and prefer to take this substance in mega doses. Taking pine pollen as a tincture works great for absorption, but it is also available in pill or powdered supplement form.

Shilajit

Pronounced sil-i-jeet, shilajit is a Sanskrit word of multiple meanings, of which the most common are "Conqueror of Mountains" and "Destroyer of Weakness." Part of the ancient Indian natural medicine system known as Ayurveda, shilajit is known as a rejuvenator and an adaptogen.

We live in a world with ever-growing stressors and fatigue attacking us from all sides. Most people fight sleep deprivation and fatigue with caffeine and sugar. You know the routine. Starbucks coffee and energy drinks—a nightmare for your adrenals. Clearly toxic coffee isn't the way to go, and sugar never helps anyone out but the bakery. What your body needs is a healthy boost, without a crash, that gives you the strength to adapt and respond in healthy ways to stress, including resisting mental and physical fatigue. This is what adaptogens like shilajit do very well.

Adaptogens are an amazing group of herbs that strengthen and improve your adrenal system's health. There are many ways to take shilajit, but it's best to avoid this herb in pill format because it's likely to contain lots of unnecessary fillers. Instead, consider taking it in powdered form with warm milk or hot water. It is also available as pure mineral pitch (resin); generally, the size of a pea dissolved in hot water is plenty for a daily serving. If taken in tonic or tincture form, up to two droppers is a full dose. Shilajit works best in conjunction with other herbs, as it increases the responses of other herbs and compounds.

Mushrooms

I'm not talking about portabella or shiitake but rather medicinal mushrooms you'll wish you had known about sooner. Cordyceps is one such mushroom, a fungus that grows on the backs of specific caterpillars throughout the high mountainous terrain of China and the low-temperature, low-oxygen Himalayas of Tibet and Nepal.

This mushroom is so widespread today because it can be reproduced in the laboratory under extremely strict conditions. When taken in conjunction with other compounds and herbs, Cordyceps has also been known to combat different aging symptoms and asthma.

Chaga is another mushroom with unique properties. Not soft like common fungi, chaga is like wood, hard and dense. It's found on trees as a growth, concentrating natural elements and compounds in order to survive. It produces rich phytochemicals, which include enzymes, sterols, and phenols. As a result, chaga has been proven to be effective against cancer cells, actually stopping them from metastasizing. It's also been documented to balance insulin and blood sugar levels, build the immune system, improve eczema, and more. Let's not forget about the energy boost you'll get with this extract, too. Chaga can be made into teas and tinctures or can be ingested a number of other ways. It's best to try this supplement in a variety of ways to find the one you prefer best.

Another favorite is the Reishi mushroom. Rich in extremely powerful antioxidant compounds, Reishi mushrooms are also used to combat cancer cells and developing tumors. Reishi mushrooms help combat free radicals within your body caused from frequent exposure to chemicals and pollutants from common household products. As with other mushrooms, Reishi mushrooms are beneficial for those suffering from asthma and other types of respiratory conditions. They have anti-inflammatory properties that help those with Alzheimer's, heart disease, and arthritis. This mushroom can be bought dried or in concentrated tablet form, capsules, and as an extract. Be careful, though—it has a very bitter taste, which can make adding it to your favorite foods not such a good idea.

Ant Extract

Right about now you might be thinking I'm crazy. Ant extract, really? Just hear me out. First, I'm not talking about your common, household ant, which has more than likely been exposed to dangerous chemicals. Instead, I'm talking about one in particular, the *Polyrhachis vicina Roger*, which has been studied in China and has been authorized by the China Ministry of Public Health to be taken as a nutritional supplement. But why would anyone want to take ant extract?

The Polyrhachis is 42% protein, containing eight of the nine essential amino acids. Containing over 20 trace minerals, including magnesium, phosphorous, iron, selenium, and zinc,

Polyrhachis can be a great addition to anyone's diet. (Trace minerals are minerals needed by the human body but in extremely small amounts.)

Just as mushrooms are heralded to improve longevity, so is the Polyrhachis taken to promote long life, increase vitality, and improve blood and circulation. This ant extract is also known to increase fertility, aid in better quality sleep, calm tension throughout the body, and strengthen the musculoskeletal system. It also increases performance in the bedroom, being a sex booster and aphrodisiac.

Another great benefit to taking ant extract is the amount of trace zinc it contains. The Polyrhachis has the greatest amount of zinc out of all living organisms. Zinc is needed for strength, muscle contraction, and many different sexual functions.

Usually bought in powdered form, Polyrhachis can be mixed with water (although it doesn't mix well with cool water), juice, or blended into a delicious ant shake.

Ashwagandha

Ashwagandha is a plant whose roots and berries are used to make tinctures and powder. It's used for arthritis, sleep troubles, anxiety, tumors, asthma, fibromyalgia, liver disease, and issues associated with menstruation. This plant is also another adaptogen, strengthening the body's response against stress. It shouldn't be used by pregnant women, though. Although no human trials have been carried out, this herb has been known to cause abortions in animals when administered in large doses.

The name for this plant is another Sanskrit word meaning "horse-like." This is likely attributed to its strong smell. Either way, with chemicals that can help calm your brain, reduce swelling, and lower your blood pressure, this is an herb you're sure to want to look into more.

Eleuthero

Another adaptogen, Eleuthero, full name *Eleutherococcus senticosus*, is known for its performance enhancing abilities for athletes. As with other herbs, research and studies have yielded incredible results.

I keep stressing adaptogens' ability to improve your body's reaction to stress. That's because stress affects us on two levels: mentally and physically. On the mental level, we may get short tempered and take our frustrations out on everyone around us. We may procrastinate and withdraw, refusing to acknowledge or deal with the stress head-on. The physical level is how your body responds to stress. This is where diseases like fibromyalgia come from. Your body may feel sore to the touch, although there aren't any signs of tenderness or injury. Your body can feel weak or fatigued. It can also have trouble relaxing under tension, which means difficulty relaxing and sleeping at night. How your body reacts to stress often amplifies how you respond to stress. That's why adaptogens are amazing supplements for your body to receive.

Athletes rely heavily on their bodies to pull through during often extremely stressful times. As a result, many turn to Eleuthero because of its ability to modulate stress, improve memory, and prevent fatigue. It builds your blood and your body's use of oxygen so your muscles get what they need during muscle-building workout sessions. Eleuthero also helps support autoimmune function.

He Shou Wu

This herb comes from the roots of *Polygonum multiflorum*, a plant native to the mountains of southern and central China. He Shou Wu is used to bring healing and restoration to the kidney and liver. Others have even seen their natural hair color restored from gray when using this powerful tonic. Weak knees and lower back pain are often signs of reduced kidney strength and performance, including low sex drive and weak sexual energy. He Shou Wu has been proven to improve performance and function in these areas, improving overall disease and injury resistance, as well as strengthening stamina and endurance, and lowering cholesterol levels.

Boasting more claims to improve sex life and energy, He Shou Wu contains components that help relieve backaches, chronic bruising, and knee joint pain. It contains anti-inflammatories, leucoanthocyanidins (LAC), which can help reduce swelling around joints, bones, and other areas that are known to cause chronic pain and stiffness.

Hydrilla

This water plant used to be a staple in many household fish tanks. However, stores had to stop selling it due to the fact that when flushed down the toilet along with dead fish, this plant would grow so quickly as to invade and infest entire ecosystems. Hydrilla has one of the most concentrated sources of vitamin B12. That means it's a great supplement for vegans and vegetarians. Meat-eaters have even been known to be low on B12, so it's beneficial for them as well.

Vitamin B12 is crucial for brain development and cell degeneration prevention, as well as overall central nervous system health. It is crucial for the formation of neurotransmitters, which your cells need in order to receive and send signals throughout your nervous system, and the myelin sheath, a keen component to your cells' reception of input and output signals.

Let me put it like this: your brain releases neurotransmitters, or chemicals, that when administered in their proper amounts communicate important information throughout your body. When these neurotransmitters are too low or too high, your mood, sleep, weight, and concentration abilities can be severely affected. Because of this, hydrilla can help alleviate struggles with depression (often affected by low levels of the neurotransmitter serotonin), fatigue, and anxiety.

You can get this plant in dried powder to mix in water. It doesn't have much of a taste, so feel free to drop it into your smoothies too if you like.

Maral Root

I love this herb because it has a great story behind it. It's known by a number of names, but the most common, Maral root, comes from the Maral deer who first turned people on to its incredible capabilities. During mating season, male deer fight for the right to mate. Afterwards, they dig the roots of the *Rhaponticum*, *Leuzea*, and *Stemmacantha carthamoides* plants up in order to restore their strength and energy. This plant has been documented to help people recover from fatigue, increase sexual drive, as well as treat impotence, alleviate mild depression, improve memory abilities, and increase work capacity.

This root also has adaptogenic properties, which make it another go-to if you're looking to improve your body's overall functioning ability. Its anabolic properties aid the body in developing lean muscle mass as well. You need to be careful if choosing to take this supplement, however, because it can increase your risk of bleeding, which can cause severe problems when taken in conjunction with other medicines.

Nettle Root

This plant is often referred to as the stinging nettle. That's due to the fine hairs located on its leaves that can cause burning pain that can last from hours to weeks. This dark green, well-protected plant can be used to treat urination issues caused by an enlarged prostate. These issues include frequent urination, nighttime urination, painful urination, irritable bladder, urinary tract infections (UTI), urinary tract inflammation, and the inability to urinate. It's also used as a diuretic and astringent, and for joint ailments.

This plant can also help optimize your hormones, like testosterone, so that you get the maximum benefit. It's not enough to have high testosterone because studies have proven that testosterone can be inhibited and in some cases even converted to estrogen by aromatization. This is where nettle root can save the day, as it is a natural aromatase inhibitor.

Guduchi

Also known as *Tinospora cordifolia*, Guduchi is considered among the top herbs in Ayurvedic medicine. This is another herb that possesses anti-inflammatory components and is thus great for arthritis. It supports the immune system and improves liver and kidney function. Various parts of this plant have produced incredible benefits for various medicinal purposes.

Oil from the Guduchi plant can be used to reduce pain, edema, gout, and different skin diseases. The taste of Guduchi is known to be bitter and sweet, pungent and astringent. It has heating action, which makes it very effective in reducing swelling in joints. Some caution is needed for diabetic patients, as it can lower blood sugar levels. Pregnant and breastfeeding women should avoid this as well since not enough studies have proven it to be safe for them.

This herb comes in powder and pill form. I tend to prefer powdered forms of many supplements, simply because of the amounts of fillers that tend to be present in encapsulated plants.

Rhodiola

Another powerful adaptogen, Rhodiola grows naturally in the harsh environment of the dry, low temperature, high altitudes of various parts of Europe, Asia, and Alaska. Not only does Rhodiola improve the body's resistance to stress, but it also improves attention, cognitive ability and function, and mental performance under prolonged stress and fatigue.

Traditionally, the plant's flowers were used to make a tea. It's rich, succulent leaves and shoots have also been boiled down and cooked like spinach, or even eaten raw. The roots contain the medicinal properties. The main claim of this powerful herb is its energy boosting capability along with its ability to improve attention span, productivity, and mood. Rhodiola extract is available in liquid or capsulations as well as ground powder.

Schisandra

Schisandra chinensis is a bright red berry of a climbing vine found in the northeast regions of China, as well as various parts of Russia. This berry also has the name of Wu Wei Zi, or five-flavored berry, because it has the taste of sweet, sour, bitter, pungent, and salty. This berry has been known traditionally to prolong life and aid in aging gently and gracefully, as well as being an energy booster, fatigue lifter, and sex booster. In addition to these radical claims, it is also a powerful antioxidant that possesses anti-inflammatory capabilities.

This herb can be combined with other herbs but should be used with caution when used in combination with other medicines. Again, pregnant and breastfeeding women should avoid this herb until more studies have been conducted to determine its safety. Because of its astringent properties, taking this herb while sick with either the common cold or flu should be avoided. Schisandra tends to hold moisture inside the body.

Schisandra is a great herbal supplement if you need your liver detoxed, have soreness or stiffness in your joints, or need a boost to your mental performance.

Triphala

This name literally means "three fruits," as it consists of three fruits used in traditional Ayurvedic medicine in order to achieve incredible results: Amalaki (*Emblica officinalis*), Bibhitaki (*Terminalia belerica*), and Haritaki (*Terminalia chebula*). This herb is known to provide the most complete form of protection for the body's main organs, including the heart, skin, and eyes. These three fruits combined can cleanse the colon, protect your liver and keep it healthy, and rid the body of dangerous toxins that can leech energy away after even the simplest of tasks.

Triphala can also safely regulate your digestive system and even improve your body's absorption ability. This herb's cleansing capabilities are best achieved through use in its powdered form. Tablets are still a good choice, as they contain the perfect dosing of the powder. If you can stomach the taste, you can make a tea out of the powder; it's a little easier on your wallet this way.

This can be mixed with juice or water, although I will caution that it has an extremely strong taste that may take some getting used to. This powder is traditionally used to cleanse the body. If you plan to use the herbal mixture for more than 100 days, it'd be best to lower your dosage after a while.

L-Glutamine

Glutamine is found and produced within your body naturally. However, after injury or intense exercise, this amino acid is likely to be in shortage. This protein is essential for removing waste from your body in the form of excess ammonia, which is a common waste product of a functioning body. It's also necessary for normal and healthy brain function, as well as digestion. Taking a supplement of L-Glutamine can help prevent or minimize muscle breakdown, as well as improve protein metabolism and synthesis (how fast protein is created within your body).

L-Glutamine can help aid stomach ulcers, stop or prevent diarrhea, and even repair "leaky gut" syndrome. It is the only amino acid that contains two amine groups. This unique property enables it to "drop" or "give up" one of the amine groups in order to combine with glucose to make n-acetylglucosamine, which is absolutely essential to repairing the lining of the intestinal wall.

It can also make acetyl-d-glucosamine upon dropping one of its amine groups, which can heal cartilage, damaged tendons, and ligaments. You can see why bodybuilders and athletes see this protein supplement as an absolute must to their daily routine.

Green Tea Extract

I previously mentioned the benefits of green tea in the Biohacking chapter. However, if you're not much of a tea drinker, and coffee isn't really your thing either, you're still in luck because an extract of green tea is always available to you as a supplement. Scientific studies have even shown that green tea extract promotes fat oxidation beyond what caffeine can produce. It carries high amounts of polyphenols and possesses strong antioxidant properties.

Green tea extract is also a viable alternative to tea bags because of the amount of concentrated tea per drop. Tea bags don't always contain the green tea goods in their entirety. In fact, many commercial forms of tea fill the bag with garbage leftovers—you know, the dust after the better-quality leaves have been sifted out. You can use extract to make your tea last longer, as most vials can last up to a month or longer depending on how many cups you have a day. Drop the liquid tea into your milk or other favorite drink, and you'll still reap the benefits.

Fermented Cod Liver Oil/Butter Oil Blend

People have been known to take each of these separately, but new research has revealed that when taken together, the blend helps establish and maintain a natural, healthy fatty acid balance within your body.

Butter that is high in vitamins contains an omega-6 fatty acid known as arachidonic acid (AA), while cod liver is potent in the omega-3 fatty acid eicosapentaenoic (EPA). The saturated fatty acids of butter oil support and sustain the efficient and effective utilization of the unsaturated fatty acids of cod liver oil. By itself, butter contains important vitamins like vitamins E, K, and CoQ enzymes. Cod liver oil contains abundant amounts of vitamins D and A.

People have reported various positive reactions to taking such a blend, while others have reported nothing at all. My guess is that the latter aren't properly monitoring their diets or keeping an adequate record of their thoughts and feelings throughout the day in relation to what they've been eating. These supplements all have incredible reputations that are well worth the research and a good trial period once you know what you're looking for a boost in.

Supplement Recap:

I cannot stress the importance of a food and supplement diary. The purpose of taking these supplements isn't to make you sound like you're more in tune with your body. After all, none of these mean anything if you don't see improvement within yourself. The goal of a proper renovation of yourself is to feel incredible and to have more energy to pursue the things you love with the time that you have.

I'm convinced that some of these supplements will help you experience just that. You might need to try a new supplement for one to three months while keeping a close, accurate diary to ensure that the results you see are real. In the end, though, I know it'll all be worth it.

Chapter 6

Summary

One of the things that I've always loved about health and fitness is the science that backs it up and leveraging that science to biohack our way to a better body, brain, and lifestyle. I know it would be nice to have a checklist like many fitness sites present that you can follow to magically and easily look and feel the way you've always dreamed about. The reality, however, is that our bodies just don't respond that way. We need precision, which is why I highly recommend getting your labs done and analyzed with my associate Dr. Anthony Beck. You can learn more about Dr. Beck by visiting <u>dranthonygbeck.com</u>.

In this book, we've covered gene regulation, which is how your body naturally regulates how genes are expressed through each period and stage of development during life. We also covered genetic switches, going into great detail about the different factors that determine how proteins transcribe and translate the code to produce more protein. In chapter two, I provided you with a detailed list of vitamins that cause DNA methylation, which is a biochemical process necessary to protein synthesis that causes the addition of a methyl group to DNA nucleotides. To wrap it all up, I addressed the issues everyone wants to know about: fat loss, muscle gain, and gene expression. We talked about satellite cells as the main source and cause for muscle growth, and then we finished by discussing how fat is burned and what happens when gene expression gets in the way. In this last section, I described how the body functions so you can see how protein synthesis is used in everything we do. Gene expression is so much a part of our lives there is no way you can talk about fitness without including the risks and side effects of the other.

As always, the information I present is to help you learn more about your body and what works for you. When it comes to determining whether or not your fitness program is working for you, I challenge you to take the following fitness test. It's been adapted from a previous article I've written based on Dr. Cobb's thoughts from Z-Health:

Fitness Test

How do you look?—Are you looking better? Are you losing weight, getting thinner, softer, harder? This is a trap I find many people falling into. Their workouts consist of so much cardio that they lose some weight, alright, and muscle goes right out with the baby and bathwater, too. If you're not liking the way your body is shedding weight, bring this up to your trainer and discuss ways to tone your body in the ways you'd like.

Troubleshooting tip: Check your temperature daily, preferably first thing upon wakening and in the early afternoon. If your temperature is consistently below 98 degrees and you see a downward trend, this is indicative of a slow metabolism. Check with your doctor of naturopathy to see if you have specific nutrient deficiencies and as a result have hypothyroidism (or another metabolic issue). I mention hypothyroidism because I believe it is often underdiagnosed. Hypothyroidism is typically diagnosed when your TSH (thyroid stimulating hormone) level reaches 4 but can actually be indicated at a TSH of 1.

How do you feel?—When I read articles about fitness, I constantly come across this one staple of encouragement for pursuing exercise: beta-endorphins. Your body releases these chemicals that are equivalent to a drug's high effect. You might have heard it referred to as the "runner's high." Maybe that's why you decided to pursue exercise—you wanted to benefit from the feel-good let down of your brain. But do you really feel better? If your exercise isn't repairing the health of your body (joints, tissues, etc.), you need to rethink what you're doing. Are you exercising with improper form? While there is some soreness that comes with building new muscle, this is only temporary and shouldn't get worse over time. Ignoring the progression of your body's health can prove fatal. Make sure you know where your body is headed.

Troubleshooting Tip: If you constantly feel sore, you may be deficient in minerals such as zinc or magnesium. You may also need to increase your intake of potassium, salt, carbohydrates, and saturated fat. All of these vitamins, minerals, and macronutrients play vital roles in muscular development and the subsequent recovery process.

How's your performance?—Exercise does more than just improve the look and feel of your body. When done correctly, it should also boost your performance across all levels to include your mental capacity at work and emotional endurance to stress at work and at home.

Troubleshooting Tip: Are you foggy headed at work and absent-minded at home? If so, check both your temperature and pulse rate. If you see your baseline levels are plummeting (i.e. resting temperature decreasing and resting pulse rate increasing), it's time to take a break. Remember, exercise is a drug that requires only a minimum effective dose, so you may need to add a deload week at the end of each month where you reduce your overall training volume, incorporate blood flow occlusion training (you can learn more about occlusion training at www.BFRBands.com), and increase your overall consumption of food (namely, carbohydrates, saturated fats, and salt).

Are you more injury-resistant?—Exercise, health, and proper nutrition heal your body. They beef up its defense systems and supercharge your immune system. While participating in your program, you should see improvements in these areas. If what you're doing seems to be making you weaker and more susceptible to injury and sickness, again, that's a sign that something is broken.

Troubleshooting Tip: If your joints are starting to feel achy, you experience a string of injuries, or your body just feels "broken," you need to consider my previous tip about overtraining. It's very easy to overlook signs of overtraining, especially in a world where more seems better, but if you're the type of person that gets anxious, moody, or even ill from missing a day at the gym, there's a high likelihood that your brain's addiction centers have become chemically hooked to the endorphins (and other morphine-like substances) released from exercise. I'm not kidding; this is very real and more common than you think. When in doubt, listen to your body and take it easy that day/week. Like I alluded to earlier, blood flow occlusion training can be very valuable here because it can expedite the recovery process by creating a bolus of blood and nutrients in the exercised tissues (and even the tissues near the exercised areas).

Closing Thoughts

I've dedicated myself to fitness. For my wife and I, our work is more than pursuing a certain look or status among our peers and friends. It's about pursuing truth and uncovering lies and misconceptions that have kept so many people from seeing the results they've been looking for for the majority of their lives. If you want to lose weight, I want to help you do it the healthy and right way.

I got into personal training first because I loved fitness. Pretty soon, however, I realized that there was a great need for accurate information. Many people just didn't know. They subscribed to popular fitness magazines and even bought into weight-loss pills and metabolism boosters only to have the same issues creep back on them: weight gain.

As you embark on your journey towards achieving optimal fitness, I can only hope that my work and research can help guide you. Keep in touch and feel free to drop me a line about whatever your goals arc. I want to help you reach them.

Join Us!

This book was brought to you by the creators of Exerscribe, a company dedicated to the biohacking movement. What is biohacking? Contrary to popular belief, hacking is about creating the shortest path to success through optimization. Biohacking is about reaching new limits, maximizing your true potential, and becoming "superhuman." No longer can we solely rely on the information from doctors or the FDA. It's our responsibility to gain the highest level of truth for our health and wellness by getting the best information possible—information that has no hidden agendas. Join our biohacking revolution and subscribe to our newsletter at exerscribe.com today. No spam or scams, you have our word.

Thank You

Thank you for reading this book. I sincerely hope the philosophies contained within have a positive impact on your life the way they have mine and many others. Please take a moment to share your thoughts with me about the book by leaving a review on Amazon. This will not only help me in future writings, but also help get this book into the hands of others. Thank you again.

About the Author

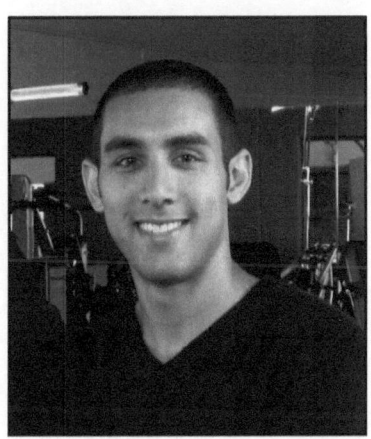

"Biohacking is the next evolution of health & fitness."

In 2006, Kusha Karvandi left his hometown of Beaverton, Oregon, for sunnier climes. He had just finished his first year at University of Oregon and decided to move San Diego. Shortly after enrolling in UC-San Diego's pre-med program, he got a side job as a personal trainer. And then the magic happened. Like most nineteen-year-olds, he had no idea what he really wanted to do with his life, but within six months he knew he had found his real passion. And it wasn't medicine.

The company he was working for at the time had gone through a reorganization, and through some stroke of luck, he managed to get a promotion to Personal Training Manager. Thanks to a few great mentors, he began mastering the nuances of both business and personal training.

After traveling across the country to run clubs in various markets, he finally had an epiphany—**why weren't gym members provided with a roadmap to success?**

Based on the principles of biohacking—achieving maximal results in minimal time—his App, Exerscribe, provides a roadmap to working out, while his books serve to change the way you eat by eliminating useless fad diets, food logging, and calorie counting. So join Kusha at exerscribe.com today and start biohacking your way to your full potential!